PRAISE FOR THIS BOOK

"I have personally benefited from putting Skip's strategies into place and feel that every other reader will too!"

Dr David Hamilton PhD,
How Your Mind Can Heal Your Body

"Skip is a force of nature and is the real deal to learn from."

Wim Hof, "The Ice Man"

"He's such an interesting guy, with an experience of magnitude. He educated me, helped me lose my belly, got me fit, made my skin better, got my jawline back, stopped me smoking and got me focused. I was in a dark place in my career, relationships and within both my mind and body... and Skip really helped me turn all these areas around. Now I am really loving life. I can't thank him enough."

Tamer Hassan, TV & movie star

"Skip is so inspirational – a great wave of energy... with his powerful, inspiring supercharged content (about) healthy exercise, nutrition, mind-set and all the rest. It's life-changing."

**Rachel Elnaugh, businesswoman,
former investor on BBC's *Dragons' Den***

"Skip saves lives, transforms lives, extends lives. His principles are simple. I consider him one of the few enlightened human beings I've met. It's been a gift having him in my life. Welcome Skip into your life, everyone will thank you for it."

**Joel Bauer, top US persuasion guru,
known as the "Mentor's Mentor"**

LIVING FOREVER YOUNG

The 10 Secrets to Optimal Strength, Energy & Vitality

Skip Archimedes

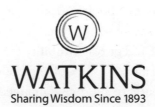

WATKINS
Sharing Wisdom Since 1893

ABOUT THE AUTHOR

Skip Archimedes is an empowering and transformational holistic health coach, motivational mentor and international speaker. Having overcome serious illness, a family break-up, obesity and depression to become a Gymnastics Champion, he then, at the age of 18, broke his back during a training session. Specialists said he would never walk again, but, unwilling to accept this, Skip went on a mission to find a cure. With intensive research, he had returned to full fitness and gained the English Sports Acrobatics Championships title within 18 months. However, he now had a wealth of knowledge about health and vitality from the best in the business in both the East and the West – and, most importantly, the power of the right mindset.

Now 45, he dedicates his life to helping people worldwide step into this same positive space, overcoming adversities, whether physical, emotional or spiritual, and living "forever young". For more information, go to: www.skiparchimedes.com

PUBLISHER'S NOTE

AUTHOR DEDICATION

I would like to dedicate this book to my wonderful mother who has always been there for me – with love, support, guidance and a belief that something great is always on the other side of every challenge. Without her, I would not have learned what I've learned and be both living forever young and helping others around the world to be doing the same.

It's been the greatest gift to be able to get my Mum to be living forever young too. There was a time when she was overweight, with high cholesterol, low blood pressure, having a lot of operations and not even that mobile, never mind feeling up to many adventures in life. And now she's got a dog that she walks every day, she swims about 100 lengths a day, and in the past 18 months alone she's been walking with lions, riding elephants and swimming with dolphins.

As somebody in her 70s, she is absolute proof that it's never too late to start your journey to living forever young. Mum, I love you so much.

This edition first published in the UK and USA 2018 by
Watkins, an imprint of Watkins Media Limited
19 Cecil Court
London WC2N 4EZ

enquiries@watkinspublishing.com

1 3 5 7 9 10 8 6 4 2

Designed and typeset by JCS Publishing Services Ltd

Printed and bound in the United Kingdom

A CIP record for this book is available from the British Library

ISBN: 978-1-78678-136-9

www.watkinspublishing.com

CONTENTS

FOREWORD

I first met my friend Skip in London at an event with Dr John D Martini and Dr David Hamilton, and I saw him energize an audience like very few people can do. This is a gift not many share and I knew he would go on to do great work around the world.

We got to know each other and bonded like great brothers. Like myself, he has dedicated his life to making a difference and helping people wherever he goes.

Skip is really authentic and amazing, truly speaking from his heart, so I encourage you to check out the "living forever young" lifestyle that he has developed and encapsulated within this book. We call him "The Miracle Man" because he has come back from excruciating defeat all the way to becoming a champion several times in his life. When someone bounces back like this, they can teach you things they have learned on their journey that you can normally only learn by walking that path yourself.

Skip walks his talk, he is a lot of fun and, by applying the techniques contained within this book, he will leave you with an empowering vision and feeling in your body unlike anything you're likely to have experienced before.

Although he often works with celebrities and top CEOs, what he is sharing are forgotten truths that will be invaluable to absolutely anyone, as they are insights into many areas of life that are needed more than ever in today's busy modern world.

I love hanging out with him, we have shared many adventures together and I really feel like it's worth experiencing some of his magic. He is a world-class coach and I have no doubt that by reading this book, you will learn things about yourself, life and others that will open you up to a lifestyle where you can reap the many varied benefits of truly "living forever young", from experiencing more joy in your every-day experiences to feeling generally more energetic, lighter and full of zest for life.

Skip is the real deal and I'm excited for you that you have this book to read because it holds many powerful secrets that you can unlock and bring into your life. And if you ever get the chance to go to one of his live events, then you'll be in for an even bigger treat because you'll experience his magic at an even deeper level.

I'm signing this off from Sacred Precincts in Hawaii, and I'm wishing you the best day ever,

David "Avocado" Wolfe

Author, adventurer, organic and biodynamic farmer, environmentalist, nutritionist and herbalist

Also US spokesperson for the Nutribullet and co-founder of *TheBestDayEver* online health magazine

INTRODUCTION

THE 10 SECRETS TO LIVING FOREVER YOUNG

Dear Friend

Congratulations on purchasing this book that I believe holds secrets that will greatly enrich your life. If you follow my suggestions, by the time you finish reading you'll be feeling and looking remarkably younger, and enjoying a more focused, energized life.

What qualifies me to know all this? In short, conquering challenge. I have been a top-level gymnast and now work around the world as a successful holistic health coach and motivational speaker but, not that long ago, I faced challenges in my life that I thought would break me. However, through digging deep, I've learned that if I face my challenges and don't back away from them — and even learn to recognize them as disguised gifts of empowerment — I can emerge stronger, better, healthier and with even more energy.

When I was a young kid I fell into a coma with pneumonia. I was covered with eczema, suffered chronic asthma and chest infections, and was nearly always on medication. Doctors told me that I shouldn't do any exercise, because I kept having asthma attacks, but a family friend — who was also asthmatic and was a gymnastics coach — disagreed. His mum ran a swimming club and they both firmly believed in the benefits of exercise, at the appropriate level, to improve anyone's health. They had seen and experienced this first hand on so many occasions. On their advice I started basic swimming and gymnastics, and very quickly the worst of my problems fell away. I found myself doing gymnastics everywhere I went. I didn't have that much natural talent compared with some of the others kids, but being active in this way made me feel really good, so I kept doing it. I started competing and, before long, I started to get better, so much so that my coaches suggested that I could go on to compete at the very highest level. My life was amazing. Then, when I was 11, my mother left my father for my gymnastics coach and I wasn't allowed to do gymnastics anymore.

Many of my health problems came back, my emotions were all over the place, and I became overweight. I hated my life and was in a sad, dark and lonely place. When I turned 18, though, I decided to take charge of my life – to lose the weight and to go back to gymnastics. I just knew it was the right thing to do. It had been years since I had practised, and I needed more strength, more balance, more flexibility and better techniques. It was a huge struggle, but I was persistent and my efforts were paying off. Then, one day about six months later, I was training with my coach and working on the high bar when I had an accident and broke my back. Doctors and specialists said I would never walk again.

I spent six months in traction in the hospital. I went to an even darker place than I'd ever been in before. For four months I was pretty unreachable but my mum, my rock, didn't give up and, one day, told me she had found out about the story of Bruce Lee – US martial artist turned actor – who had broken his back, but had refused to accept his diagnosis. Instead, he set out to defy doctors and experts and he came back stronger and fitter than before. He gave me hope. I started to study Lee's philosophy for life (he died in 1973) and the philosophies of the people who inspired him, such as Confucius and the Buddha. I devoured everything I could about these inspirational figures and started to explore the power of the mind, body and spirit through both Eastern and Western approaches. Before I knew it, a world I hadn't even known existed opened up before me. My connection to life changed and I started believing anything was possible.

When I changed, everything else in my life changed too. Without it making any sense to the experts around me, I was able to stand again. That's when I learned true gratitude, because when you think you're never going to stand again and then you do, you appreciate it so much more. That soon led to me taking my first steps again. Even as I write, I can feel the emotions of that time flooding through me. Over the following weeks and months, bit by bit, I started walking, climbing, jumping, running and, before I knew it, I was independent again.

My mother then asked me what I wanted to do with my life. If the experience of breaking my back had taught me anything, it was how important it is to do what you love. Well, I loved gymnastics. Even though it was through practising gymnastics that I'd been to the darkest places possible, and logically it should be the last thing I'd want to do again, Bruce Lee's philosophy had taught me – don't think, feel. I went back to gymnastics and within two years of training with a double World Champion, together we won the English Sports Acrobatics Championship title. Why am I telling you all this? Because no matter how you are challenged – or how tired, unwell or lacking in energy you feel right now – you can rise up higher and stronger than before. And I'm going to give you the secrets as to how.

ABOUT THIS BOOK

Let me be clear right from the start: this book is neither an exercise book nor a nutrition book, although both of those subjects come up. It is more of a life-enhancement book. Through it, I'll guide you along your life's path so that you can reach for more fulfilment and more success in both a mind and body that will feel younger and more vibrant than before.

This book is about transforming your life in ten key ways in order to improve how you look and feel every day, while also enhancing your longevity so that you get to spend more time with those you love. It's about helping you to recognize that while we all, of course, get older, we don't have to feel and act "old" in the way that Western society most often predicts – feeling sick, tired, weak and frail. Instead, we can choose to live healthily, really "grow" older and feel "forever young".

When I talk about "living forever young", it's not about getting on board with the latest fad or trend. And neither is it in any way trying to reject blindly the fact that we all get older (and, if we're lucky, wiser!). Living forever young simply involves exploring and putting into practice a lifestyle that really serves *you*, no matter what age or life stage you're at. You might be a student, an entrepreneur, a parent, a grandparent or anyone in between – wherever you are in life, my techniques will work for you, because they are accessible and can be personalized according to your own situation. Take my secrets and make them your own.

The ten "secrets" of living forever young in this book might at first glance not seem like secrets at all – until, that is, you recognize that even though you may already know a lot of the things in theory, you aren't actually "living" them. The real "secret", therefore, is in me helping you figure out how to use the information in this book for *yourself*. This is not about drowning you in more information, but instead helping you to tap into the wisdom you were born with, but have forgotten along life's path.

You'll learn that you really can take something from your mind and pull it into your reality. You'll also learn how to free your mind from stress and get the most from your body, achieving more strength, balance and flexibility. And you'll learn the greatest secret of all: how to play with life, so that you live with the boundless energy and wonder that you had as a child, when the world had endless possibility.

I believe that we are living at the best time in human history – we are learning, creating, evolving faster than ever before. And yet, I feel like we've forgotten how to live our lives to the full, because there is so much disease, illness, depression, crime and negativity around us. By living the ten secrets that I have chosen from my years of experience exploring health and wellness, I believe you'll experience more of what you really want from life (whatever that may be) and feel both happy and "successful" – by being truer to yourself and your passions, and finding a stronger sense of purpose and belief in life.

The ten "secrets" that I have identified as empowering us to live in the most vibrant, "forever young" way are:

- Breathe: enjoying lovely, full, healthy breathing.
- Move: ensuring that you fit plenty of activity and exercise into your daily life.
- Nourish: making healthy choices about what you eat, drink and absorb on an emotional level.
- Rest: treating yourself to lots of quality rest and recuperation.
- Love: living with kindness and compassion in abundance, both towards yourself and others.
- Shine: bathing in the light of the sun and shining your own radiance out into the world.
- Believe: having faith and belief in your deepest self and living a life that is true to that identity.
- Learn: embracing new ideas and experiences that nurture your mind and allow you to evolve as a person.
- Commit: approaching everything you undertake with resilience and conviction.
- Live: surrounding yourself with positive energy and creating an environment that celebrates your individuality and nurtures your sense of purpose.

The beautiful thing about enhancing these ten key areas of your life is that no matter what stage you are at with things, there is always another level to reach, so there's always room to grow no matter how well or happy you already feel.

Nothing in life tastes as good as "living forever young". My wish for you is that this book becomes your book of change. I want you to carry it around with you and revisit it many times over. Each time you come back, you'll find yourself unlocking more of the lifestyle you dream of, because its wisdom will keep being relevant to you, for the rest of your life.

RECURRING THEMES

Even though each of the ten secrets in the book is distinct, there are several important themes that recur, which are core to my teachings. It's useful to introduce these now, before you begin.

Understanding your body

As children we mostly live in our bodies – we are physical, instinctual, impulsive, natural. As adults most of us live in our minds. Throughout the book I'll be encouraging you to get out of your overly active mind and reconnecting you with the miracle of the human body.

I'll be adding some more flexibility into your life, because if the body gets stiff, not only are you less physically able than you used to be, but your mind tends to get stuck, too. Discovering ways of moving that are fun, intuitive and joyful for you will help you get back into your physical body and slow down the ageing of both your body and mind.

I also firmly believe in the benefits of an alkaline diet for optimum health – for so many people too much acidity within the body is basically rusting them from the inside out. The natural state for your body is alkaline, and when acid takes hold it speeds up ageing and can lead to all sorts of diseases. During my research, I have found men and women who are living well into their hundreds and are very active. The people I've met who live this long are very alkaline, so I believe this is key in your journey to living forever young.

Understanding your mind

Nothing in life means anything until you pin your own meaning on it. So, understanding your mind is fundamental. We'll look at improving memory and learning, but more than that we'll be looking at how to declutter your mind so that you experience more clarity in your life (I can feel you relax at the thought of that!). When the mind is clear, you can focus on making sure your thoughts are positive and serve you, rather than being negative and stressful. Your mind directs your thoughts, feelings and actions – it's time to take control of it in the most positive ways possible.

Understanding your spirit

Most of us use wifi these days, right? We can't see it, touch it or smell it as it's formless – non-physical, right? Yet in daily life, we rely upon it – to the extent that when it drops off, we get stressed out as we feel completely "disconnected". This is a fantastic analogy for what we call our "spirit", the sense of soul and energy that can add so much power, belief, magic, strength, wisdom, pleasure, joy and love to our lives. If we choose not to believe in it, or if we allow ourselves to become disconnected from this "spirit", we tend to feel stressed (we might not know that's the reason, but it is).

The easiest and most natural way to reconnect with the spirit is simply to find and do what gives you true joy! Finding your joy opens you up to a fundamental life-force energy that lies inside of each one of us. Many of the world's ancient cultures talk about this energy living in our "subtle" or non-physical body. When this life-force energy flows freely around your subtle body, you feel happy, relaxed, at peace and in balance.

I've been lucky enough to work with some incredibly spiritual people, shamans and healers, who I believe are among the most enlightened beings alive today. They have shared with me ancient and timeless wisdom that can reconnect us and resonate within our modern lives. Where does this wisdom lie? I believe it's in the spaces in life – the spaces within our cells, in our minds, even between the words on this page. The space is where the spirit lies because it's formless and limitless. There is so much more to you, to life and to the universe than the human eye can see. Connecting with the spaces opens us up to more possibilities and helps us to see beyond fear and doubt, to a place free from worry and filled only with light, confidence, and flow.

PUTTING IT ALL TOGETHER: HOW TO USE THIS BOOK

The best way to use this book is to slowly work through each chapter in order to really understand each "secret" and how to apply it to your life. I recommend reading the secrets in order, as each builds on the one before it. There is some crossover, but persevere with each chapter and take steps to implement the ideas and exercises in your life. If, however, you're short for time and feel that a certain chapter may be of *particular* benefit to you, then by all means do dive in there as a starting point.

When you've been through the book once, read it again. Or, if you don't have time to read the whole thing, then read a chapter that you found either particularly useful or particularly challenging the first time round.

I recommend reading the book several times if possible, even if this is over a long period of time. Each time you'll discover something new, or rediscover something you'd forgotten. And reading it more than once will enable you to embed the information and properly implement it. You want the advice to become a natural, instinctual part of your life, not something you're forcing.

The first time you read it the information will come onto your radar and you will likely start taking some steps towards your goals. The second time, I believe you will feel like you are reading a different book altogether – you will see some totally new and different things in it that you missed the first time around. Keep going a few more times and the guidance within the book will really seep into your soul – you will be living it more instinctually and radiating out your new energy, youth and happiness.

What will each chapter hold in store?

At the start of each chapter I'll introduce you to that chapter's secret and give an overview of what the chapter will contain.

You'll then find a section called **"Where are you now? (Part 1)"**. This presents **five statements** relating to the secret in question, which I invite you to score on the basis of how true it is for you. Keep a note of your score in a dedicated notebook. When you respond to the statements, try not to think about them too much. Instead, just let your body feed you the score (this may sound strange, but you just need to follow your instincts – don't let mental chatter get in the way of your instinctual responses to the statements).

At the end of each chapter you'll be asked to look at the same five statements – **"Where are you now? (Part 2)"** – and score yourself again. Ideally, each time you read the chapter and implement more of the suggestions, your score will increase, so be sure to keep a note of your results. I suggest you aim for a score of 40 or more out of 50. Once you've hit a score of 40 or higher, congratulations! You're rocking that secret! And if you're score isn't yet up there, there's no need to worry. There will be some tips on how to achieve this.

But please don't panic if you haven't reached your desired score. Sometimes old patterns can take a while to break, so keep the faith and keep at it. If necessary, return to the "Over to you" section in each chapter in order to revisit your key action points – to ensure that as well as being the ones you like the *idea* of doing, they are also the ones that you feel fully confident about being able to fit into your daily comings and goings. Are they still the ones that feel the most appropriate to where you are with things right now? Then, once you have implemented your revised techniques/action points for a sustained period, try rescoring yourself again using the "Where are you now? (Part 2)" section and see how you get on this time. Little by little, you should start to both see – and *feel* – the results

In between these two chances to assess yourself, you will be given lots of valuable information, including a range of practical activities and exercises to help reinforce the chapter's main theme. For some of these activities, I have created accompanying **online resources**, too, which you will find marked with an asterisk (*) as they appear throughout the book; a full list of these resources can be found on page 227.

Each chapter also contains a list of **living forever young top 10 takeaways**. These are summary statements or reminders of ideas covered in the chapter. If you feel in need of inspiration one day and don't have time to read the whole chapter, go to these for a gentle, accessible prompt about the key principles you need to keep in mind.

Each chapter also contains at least one quote by a contemporary of mine who I find inspiring in the world of wellness. These little cherry-picked gems provide extra insight, and another perspective, on the theme in hand.

Crucially, you will also always find an **"Over to you"** section towards the end of every chapter where you will be encouraged to engage on a personal level with what you have just read in order to decide on – and commit to – the main ways in which you are going to integrate new, healthy "living forever young" habits into your daily life from today onwards.

If ever you are finding it tricky to decide what to commit to, try this **"Lost in Music"** technique to help you get out of your head and more into your heart and body:

- Put on a song that you find fun and energizing.
- Let yourself go and really feel the good vibes of the music, tuning in to the innermost feelings and instincts of your body.
- Feel free to move around, dance and even sing if you like, remembering the theme of the chapter you just read, but not focusing too intensely on it.
- When the song is finished, take a deep breath, sit down with your pen and paper and instinctively write down three small ways in which you could start to put the chapter's suggestions into practice, without overthinking it. If three feels too tough, focus on just getting one down to start with and go from there.

And, finally, you'll also find a reminder about coming back to a **life-balance wheel exercise** that I encourage my clients to do at regular intervals to assess how fulfilling the different main areas of their life feel in the present moment – in order to work out which areas could do with most time and energy devoted to them. See overleaf for more information on this.

Remember, your journey is unique and while I can guide you with the overall themes, I can't predict your journey. I will, however, provide guidance for you to help you get into the best head (and heart) space possible to choose action points that you feel able, confident and excited about genuinely implementing from that day onwards.

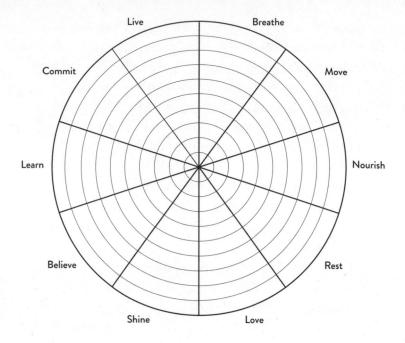

THE LIFE–BALANCE WHEEL EXERCISE

Above is an example of the life-balance wheel mentioned a moment ago. Note that each segment of the wheel corresponds to one of the chapters in this book – the 10 "secrets" of "living forever young", with the idea being that you have a chance to assess how fulfilled you currently feel in each area of your life.

Copy this wheel several times, whether by photocopier or by hand, and use one of the copies to do the exercise, rather than this original, so that you always have the blank version should you need more copies in the future.

Then take one of your copies of the wheel and go clockwise around it, starting at "Breathe" and filling in what seems right for you on a gut level in terms of how fulfilling that area of your life feels. If you feel you're already at 100 percent in any of the sections, as that area of your life feels

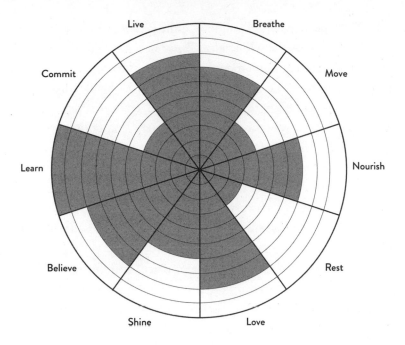

completely amazing, then you can shade in the whole of that segment. If, for example, you feel you get a lot of pretty good rest, but there's room for some improvement, you might shade 80 percent of the Rest segment. If you feel you're at 50 percent, then shade half the segment, etc. If you feel that a particular aspect is completely lacking in your life, then you don't need to fill in any of that section. And so on... Note that I'm writing "feel" because it's much more powerful to "feel" something than to just think it... Feel free to use a different colour for each segment if you are a visual thinker, but just plain old pen or pencil are fine too.

Above is an example of a wheel that has been filled in. You can see that this person feels very happy with their progress on Learn but could do with devoting more of their time to enhancing the Rest, Move and Commit aspects of their life, which means they might choose to focus on those chapters in the book first, or more than the others.

Each person's wheel will look quite different in terms of balance – that's the whole idea. But, once you've read each chapter and started implementing its tips and techniques, I invite you to take one of the other copies of the blank wheel you've made and fill in the relevant section again. Keep going as you work your way through each chapter. Then, once all ten segments are filled in, compare this version to the wheel you filled in before you started reading to see your progress.

Repeat this exercise every time you re-read a chapter or the book, marking each version with the date for your future reference. I hope this will give you a nice visual representation of your progress.

Although we'll all be at different places at different times, we all share the common goal of all the areas in our life being not only balanced but also as fulfilling, and therefore as complete, as possible.

TOP TIPS TO HELP YOU ON YOUR WAY

Finally, before you begin the "living forever young" journey, here are my top truths to help you focus and prepare.

- Don't focus on the problems in life, be solution driven and cherish your loved ones by creating magic memories.
- Material possessions won't make you happy. Choose health as your foundation.
- Don't chase happiness – become happiness and share that blessing.
- Spend time helping people – it serves your well-being.
- You'll lose yourself if you try to make everyone else happy. Instead, focus on finding happiness within you and radiate it outwards to those around you.
- Perfection doesn't exist – if you get sucked into trying to

make things perfect, you only create suffering.

- Actions always speak louder than words, so don't just think or speak – do!
- Practise your talents – they are unique and special and will make you feel good.
- Your past doesn't equal your future so learn to live in each moment.
- You are the writer, director and star of your life so make it a life worth living. You are in charge and in control over yourself (but not over anyone else).
- It's not what happens to you in life that matters, it's how you respond to and grow with what happens that counts.
- Reconnect to your inner child – become more playful, innocent, honest, inquisitive and authentic.
- Every day have a little dance like no one is watching and feel that freedom within your body and mind.
- See what's great about people, yourself and life and don't get trapped into being a part of the problem – become a part of the solution.
- As "young" as we can stay, we will all die in the end, and we don't know when: every day is a gift, so make the most if it.

Most of all – enjoy!
Live Strong, Live Healthy, Live Long & Live Now!
Skip

SECRET 1: BREATHE

When a good friend of mine told me that I couldn't tell people how to breathe, never mind set it up as a "secret" in my new book, I thoroughly disagreed. While breathing in itself is no secret, of course (we all do it automatically whether awake or asleep), the art of breathing *properly* – deeply and fully – is definitely something that most people could do with paying more attention to. The simple fact of the matter is that even if we know what's meant by "proper" breathing, very few of us actually practise it.

In this chapter I'll explain what optimal breathing really is – why it's essential, what it does and then how to do it so that it benefits your whole body, mind and spirit. We'll look at the physiology of breath and the importance of oxygen for living forever young, and along the way we'll take a look at some structured breathing techniques that will help you to get your full breath back.

But, before we begin, let's look at where you are with your breathing right now.

WHERE ARE YOU NOW? (PART 1)

Please score the following statements for your breathing on a scale of 1 to 10, with 1 being "not at all true for me" and 10 being "completely true for me". Note down your score. Then when you've completed this chapter and started implementing its advice, try the questions again.

- When I take a regular breath, my tummy pushes out before my chest.

- When I hit an obstacle in my day, I pause and take a deep breath before responding.
- I make a conscious effort to use my breath as a focus for calming meditation or me-time everyday.
- I have never had a panic attack or a feeling of tightness in my chest and lack of breath when I'm stressed.
- I am able to exercise for 30 minutes at 60 percent effort without getting out of breath.

THE NEED TO BREATHE

The human body needs lots of different nutrients, along with water and myriad metabolic processes to stay alive. But nothing is more essential to your survival than oxygen – all the cells in your body, from your toenails to your liver to your heart to your brain, need it. In fact, you need it so much that your clever body makes sure you get it even without you having to think about it.

The trouble is that because we don't have to think about breathing, many of us don't breathe properly. By "properly" I mean deep into your lungs, letting the breath push out your belly and rise up to fill your lungs and push out your chest. We all used to breathe naturally like this, as babies, but as we age most of us stop holding ourselves fully upright (check your posture now – are you hunched over?), limiting the space our lungs have to expand and reducing the amount of oxygen we breathe in on each breath. Before long, it becomes habitual to breathe using only the top part of our lungs – chest out, belly stationary.

A QUICK LESSON IN RESPIRATION

Breathing is important. Look at it this way: if you're ever stuck out in the wilderness you'll survive about three weeks without food; about three days without water; in a blizzard or blistering heat you'll need a shelter within about three hours; but – and here's the kicker – you'll live only about three whole minutes without oxygen. Before we go any further, I want to give you a quick overview of what happens when you breathe, so that you understand why it's so important for living forever young.

A single in-breath is in fact a series of muscular contractions that suck air into your lungs – your diaphragm (a belt of muscle that arcs across your torso) contracts and flattens downwards, and the muscles between your ribs (your intercostal muscles) also contract. The combination of these two actions creates a vacuum that forces air in through your nose or mouth and into your lungs. When the diaphragm and intercostal muscles relax, air is then pushed out.

Once air is inside your lungs, tiny balloon-like structures called alveoli expand, and molecules of oxygen pass through the alveoli cell walls into your blood stream. All the tiny blood capillaries around the alveoli flow into the pulmonary vein, the main blood vessel that takes blood from your lungs into your heart, from where it is pumped around your entire body – your cells giving up their oxygen to energize all your body systems. So, you see, when you breathe correctly, your whole body benefits and your energy levels are increased.

Just in case you need any more convincing, here are some research facts about breathing that I found pretty mind-blowing.

In 1923, German physiologist Dr Otto Warburg starved some rat cells of oxygen, reducing the amount of oxygen available to them by 70 percent compared with the amount they would have in a living body. Some of those cells died, some weakened and most mutated – generally, cells that mutate may become cancerous. Dr Harry Goldblatt, a US researcher well-known in the mid-1900s for his expertise in the nature of blood, made similar discoveries. On the other hand, Dr Alexis Carrel, a French biologist working in the first half of the 20th century, took cells from elderly chickens (12 years old, which in chicken years is ancient) and made sure they were fed the correct amount of oxygen. He also made sure those cells had the correct nutrients and were free from waste products. Those chicken cells, even though in chicken terms they were almost ready to die, ended up outliving Carrel himself. Before he died, he wrote, "If you give cells what they need (oxygen and nutrients, and the elimination of waste) and you avoid physical rupture, then the cells can live forever."

Just to be clear: I'm not saying that if we don't all start breathing properly, we're all going to end up desperately ill. Or that if we do start breathing better that we'll live forever. I just want to illustrate the point that breathing is fundamental, essential and life-giving. (It's also worth noting that pure oxygen treatments can be harmful to health. The best source of oxygen comes from the cleanest air you can find.)

It's a true story...

When I was a child I lived with constant chest infections and was pretty much always on some type of medication. Whenever I did any form of exercise, I would lose my breath and often have an asthma attack. The advice I was given was to do no exercise at all as exercise clearly wasn't good for me. Although I didn't realize it at the time, in fact this was the opposite of good advice! Rather, I needed to strengthen my lungs through breathing deeply during exercise, because my lungs had become weak from lack of use. As mentioned in the introduction, a friend of the family advised me to take up swimming and gymnastics to strengthen my body and my lungs and improve my overall fitness. This completely changed my life for the better. I was exercising, breathing properly and strengthening my body and my mind. My health started to improve from day one, the exercise I was doing was really fun (it's key to enjoy what you do) and it proved to be the best medicine.

Every day you need to have fresh air. Air is everything. That's the number one thing to you living.

Don Tolman, "Wholefood Medicine Man", trainer and author

LEARNING TO BREATHE AGAIN

Getting the most out of each breath is really a case of "use it or lose it" – your lungs need exercise, just like the muscles of your arms, legs, abdomen and all the rest. If you can relearn how to breathe properly, like you did when you were a child, you can strengthen your lungs, increase their capacity and make sure you're flooding your body with life-giving, health-giving oxygen that will help to keep you forever young. If you ignore the state of your breathing, you'll find that the lack of oxygen in your body can cause tiredness, fatigue and increased toxicity (bearing in mind that every exhalation is breathing out toxins, so breathing out shallowly doesn't expel as many toxins as is desirable). Lack of deep, healthful breathing will also lead to premature ageing in your skin and other cells of your body. An editorial in the *Journal of the Royal Society of Medicine* suggested that fast, shallow breathing can cause fatigue, sleep disorders, anxiety, stomach upsets, heartburn, wind, muscle cramps, dizziness, visual problems, chest pain and heart palpitations. The list is long – and unnecessarily scary!

Good breathing comes from your lower rather than upper torso. Each breath should expand your belly, your lower back and ribs. Think about filling up a glass of water. Water starts at the bottom of the glass and rises to the top.

When you breathe properly, you'll find that exerting yourself during exercise causes less shortness of breath, and you'll have greater stamina to keep going for longer.

Try it now: Three minutes of freedom*

Right now, as you breathe in, let your belly expand first, then your chest; and then as you exhale let your belly contract and push out all the stagnant air.

Now try this diaphragmatic breathing exercise, and aim to practise it for just three minutes twice a day, every day. I call it "Three Minutes of Freedom" because you're freeing up your lungs to take in life-giving oxygen, and it has a wonderful side-effect of freeing up space in your mind, too. Keep your breaths long and slow throughout, trying to make the exhale longer than the inhale. Most people take 12 to 16 breaths per minute; aim instead for eight to ten, making them deeper and more meaningful.

- Sit, lie or stand with your back straight. (You can play gentle music in the background if you like, and try to give yourself a view of nature – although that's not essential, of course.) Set a stopwatch or timer for three minutes, and begin.
- Relax your shoulders on an out-breath, noticing them drop away from your ears as you let any tension go.
- Put your hands on your stomach, fingertips touching, and take a breath in. Watch the breath moving past your chest and watch your hands on your belly rise, and your fingertips pull apart, as the breath reaches the lowest part of your lungs.
- Then breathe out, watching your hands on your belly fall as you do so. Try to make your exhale a little longer than your inhale, to ensure you've pushed out

»

all the stale air before you take the next in-breath. Remember, long, slow breaths. Pause after each exhale without taking a breath. Focus on the stillness – your body will breathe when it needs to.

- You can breathe in through your nose and out through your mouth, if you like, or both in and out through your nose if you prefer. Just choose a style that works for you. The key thing is to fill your lungs with oxygen.
- Keep breathing, watching your hands rise and fall for a full three minutes. When the three minutes are up, release your hands and take a few natural breaths, before moving on with your day.

I've found that it can take only ten minutes to teach someone to learn to breathe properly again. If you practise this exercise of breathing down into your belly twice a day for a week, however, I'm confident that proper, diaphragmatic breathing will become second nature to you again after a while. I recommend setting reminders on your phone or posting them around your home so that you remember to make time to do this exercise twice a day. Repetition and consistency are key in making this full, deep breathing automatic again.

BREATHING TO STAY FOREVER YOUNG

So, you've learned to breathe "properly" again and you know that doing so will help to keep your body's cells properly oxygenated and healthy. How does that manifest into living forever young?

Reducing toxicity

Toxins are everywhere – in your food, in the air, even in your own body as a result of stress or anxiety. Breathing not only brings life-giving oxygen into your body; it eliminates life-limiting toxins from it, too. In fact, breathing accounts for about 70 percent of your body's function to get rid of harmful toxins.

Repairing your skin cells

Oxygen enables all your body's cells to thrive (it's why people with critical injuries are often put in oxygen chambers – flooding the body and all its components with the very nutrient it needs for life). It stands to reason, then, that your skin cells need oxygen to thrive. At the deepest levels of your skin, oxygen is essential for the process that helps your skin cells manufacture collagen and elastin, which give your skin its elasticity. On the outermost levels, your skin needs oxygen for healthy cell turnover – old skin cells shedding away and being replaced with new, healthy cells that keep you blemish-free.

Releasing pain

Tension and physical pain, including headaches, and joint and muscle pain, can be relaxed and released by breathing into the pain. You can use the "Three Minutes of Freedom" exercise (see page 6) to do this – only this time, with each in-breath visualize the breath going to the place of pain and imagine this pain releasing a little each time you exhale. When we are in discomfort we often unknowingly make the mistake of holding our breath rather than breathing consciously and purposefully to let the pain go. The truth is that while there is a mental release in this practice, there is also physical release – without oxygen, your body can't repair itself.

Reducing your stress

If you've ever suffered a panic attack, you'll know that terrifying tightness that comes into your chest, as if you can't breathe.

That's because during heightened stress, your blood vessels dilate, diverting all your blood to your muscles in order to prepare you to fight or flee danger. In effect, your oxygen supply rapidly falls, breathing becomes shallow and rapid, and overall the body becomes starved of oxygen.

We can therefore use breathing to combat stress effectively, breathing deeply into our abdomen to restore a sense of calm. Try the exercise on the following page to reduce a feeling of stress and encourage relaxation and balance.

Improving self-control

Think back over the last week. How many times have you had a knee-jerk reaction that has made you lash out either by snapping at someone or slamming a door, or even just scowling at your computer screen in rage? The thing is that by reacting in one of those ways, you become part of the problem, integrated into it, rather than holding yourself outside of it so that you can resolve it.

What, then, if you used your breath to create a pause? Next time you find your emotions feeling out of control, stop what you're doing and focus on your breath. Literally just switch your attention to that feeling of an in-breath on the tip of your nose. Feel it (just like you did in the last exercise, on page 6) and allow the breath to calm you. Follow your breath in and follow your breath out. With this little bit of breath focus, you create a space between you and the problem. Once you start to notice that you're feeling a little better, which can happen in a matter of seconds, you can go back to the situation and look at it with a greater sense of balance and proportion. You are now a calm observer, rather than part of the problem, and in a much better place to find a reasonable, considered solution.

Nourishing the spirit

I love the spirit part of who we are, because when I help people to reconnect to their non-visible and non-physical aspects, they

Breathing for relaxation and balance

First, focus on your posture. Look how a child holds him- or herself: shoulders are naturally back and down; the back is naturally straight and the chest open. This is essential for proper breathing – if you're hunched over, or holding tension in your neck and shoulders, you can't possibly get proper breaths into your lungs. Relax your posture and breathe deeply. Practise the following exercise when you feel tension rising or at the end of a stressful day to restore a sense of calm. It only takes two minutes, so you definitely have time for it! Don't try to change your breath for this exercise, just notice how it feels to you.

- Sit, stand or lie comfortably somewhere where you'll be undisturbed. Focus fully on the feeling of your breath, noticing it on the tip of your nose, or on your lips as you breathe in and out. Really notice the feeling, allowing that feeling to fill your entire consciousness. Experience drawing in slow, controlled breaths, not gulping in or blowing out. Don't take control of the rhythm, just let your breathing happen.
- Now, if you aren't doing so already, breathe both in and out of your nose. Take long breaths that fill your entire belly and lungs – remember, you're not forcing the breaths, just let them happen naturally. Start to feel the rhythm of your natural breathing. As you do so, stress will naturally start to ebb away. Continue for two minutes altogether.

experience a natural state that is filled with good vibes, beyond the realm of thoughts to a place where anything is possible. During my work with the breath, I've seen people have out-of-body experiences, when they appear to be floating above themselves observing what's happening, conquer debilitating pain and even focus their eyes when previously they had needed glasses. It seems extraordinary, but it's true – and breath work is a big part of the process.

Breath brings mind, body and spirit together in harmony, raising you to a higher frequency (see page 159) and enabling you to achieve deep self-healing. Although this concept might sound unreal to us in the West, in Eastern practices the notion of the mind–body–breath connection is an essential part of spiritual and physical understanding. Take yoga, for example. Yogis believe that the body flows with a life-force energy known as *prana* (this same energy is known as *chi* in traditional Chinese medicine, and *ki* in Japanese medicine). This energy, like the energy our sun gives all life on our planet, never runs out. Yoga practitioners use what are called *pranayama* – breathing techniques – to connect the body and breath in order to free up the flow of subtle energy through the body to promote balance and good health, and to nourish the spirit. They believe it not only promotes a healthy body and mind, but lengthens life, too.

There are many forms of *pranayama*, all of which help to flood the body with oxygen through deep, rhythmic and purposeful breathing. During *pranayama*, your lungs will expand and your diaphragm will flatten. This movement of your diaphragm massages your internal organs, including your liver, stomach and kidneys, freeing up the flow of *prana* throughout your entire physiology.

I like to practise *pranayama* exercises while I'm stuck in traffic or on a plane. Of course, it improves the oxygen flow within my body, but it also provides me with a focus and a sense of calm. It strengthens my spirit – turning dead time into time that helps improve not only my physical health, but my mental health, too. For those who may experience heavy tension headaches that come on at the end of a tiring day, *pranayama* can help to relieve them.

How to practise *ujjayi pranayama*

Pranayama is not just about deep breathing; it is about learning to control the breath and, in the case below, achieving the deepest possible breathing. This will allow you to expand your lungs to their fullest capacity and to use the considered and rhythmic repetition of the breath to calm your mind:

- Sit or stand comfortably with your spine straight. When you're comfortable, breathe in deeply through your nose for as long as possible, allowing your stomach to naturally extend outwards, as if your breath were blowing your stomach up like a balloon.
- As you do this, aim to create a hollow sound in the back of your throat, a bit like the sound "Haaaaaa" but with your mouth closed. Think Darth Vader! Or, if you prefer something a little less dark, the sound of ocean waves, as this form of breathing, known in the yogic tradition as *ujjayi pranayama*, is also sometimes known as the ocean breath.
- When your stomach is at its fullest capacity, begin your exhale, again through your nose. Make the out-breath long and slow, again creating this meditative hollow sound in the back of your throat. Allow your

»

stomach to deflate, hugging your belly button in to your spine.

- Once you've set your exhalation free, breathe in fully again. Allow yourself to settle into a rhythm with the soothing in- and out-breaths of this *ujjayi pranayama* technique.

- Keep going for as long as feels good, concentrating on your breath only. If your mind wanders, simply bring it back to focus on the sound, movement and feeling of your breath. Remember that your stomach expands on the inhale and deflates on the exhale.

- Then, when you're ready, simply relax back into your normal breathing.

Buddhist monk Thich Nhat Hanh has said, "Without full awareness of breathing, there can be no development of meditative stability and understanding." As in yoga, so in Buddhism there is the connection between mind, body, spirit and breath. Through the breath we have a channel to still the mind and give our life-force energy the space it deserves to flourish and flow freely. We develop compassion, love and understanding for ourselves and the world around us.

BREATHING OUTSIDE

There is no doubt that breathing deeply outside when you are surrounded by nature will make you feel more alive. Breathing deep lungfuls of good, clean air – be this in your garden or a park, in a forest, by the sea or anywhere else in the natural world – is the best way to flood your body's cells with oxygen and maximize all of the benefits of good breathing that we've discussed. If you struggle to get outside for any reason and working on your breath inside a building is your only option, don't worry, you will still benefit from the breathing exercises and from breathing more fully, but being outside as much as you can is the optimum environment for this work.

NOW YOU CAN BREATHE

Now that you have relearned what you could always do naturally as a child, you should be able to breathe for better lung strength, better organ health, managed pain, improved skin, a calmer mind and a greater connection to your spirit, all of which should leave you feeling lighter, more energized and, of course, younger! Furthermore, you will have learned to use your breath in times of stress, to create a pause, help centre yourself, and create an environment where you can respond kindly and with compassion – for yourself, the circumstances and anyone else involved – in any situation.

LIVING FOREVER YOUNG
TOP 10 TAKEAWAYS: BREATHE

- Think of your breath as a means to cleanse your body, removing toxins with each out-breath.
- Integrate exercise and movement into your life whenever possible to improve your breath – when your lungs become stronger, your breath becomes stronger, too.
- Breathe outside – enjoy fresh air as often as you can.
- Use your breath as a focus – allowing you to still the mind and concentrate on the moment in hand.
- Improve your posture and so your breath – sit or stand tall,

roll your shoulders down and back, and open your chest and torso, so that your breath can be deep and sustaining.

- Breathe into your belly and allow the breath to fill up to your chest – as if you were filling a glass of water, from bottom to top.
- Practise *pranayama* as often as you can (see an example on page 11) as a way of strengthening your breath and also as a massage for your internal organs.
- Also think of your *pranayama* as a chance to enhance your energy and to increase the harmony between your body, mind and spirit.
- Let go of any pain using the power of your breath – imagine pain releasing with each out-breath.
- Use your breath to improve your self-control – pause, breathe, act.

OVER TO YOU

Now that you've read the bulk of this chapter, it's time for you to choose how exactly you are going to make the secrets of good breathing *your own* by integrating them into your daily life. So...

- Close the book and consider the ways in which you would feel most able and happy to start putting this chapter's suggestions, or any other breathing-related ideas of your own that you have, into practice.
- Then take a pen and notebook or piece of paper and write down the three, or five, of these ways that you most like the idea of really committing to, and that you feel will not only be really useful for you, but also achievable and sustainable. For example, you might commit to practising a breathing exercise every day at a set time, such as when you first

wake up; schedule a regular date with the great outdoors; or set an app on your phone to remind you to check you are breathing to your full capacity at regular intervals throughout the day.

- If the thought of three or five things overwhelms you, just start with one – baby steps are the best way to go and as long as you keep up what you have started you'll soon find momentum building and you will want to, and be able to, do more.

- If you need a little help and encouragement to get into this decision-making zone, try the "Lost in Music" technique on page xxi of the Introduction to set you on your way.

- Then read your chosen action points out loud to yourself – and make an inward commitment about how, when and where you're going to start putting them into practice – as of this week, or even *today* if possible. Feel free to write these practical details beneath the action points if you feel it will help you stick at them…

- Now use this list as your personal guide to enhancing the "Breathe" section of your life-balance wheel, coming back to the list any time you feel the need to revise it or add to it…

✎

WHERE ARE YOU NOW? (PART 2)

Once you have been using the above list of action points for about a month, it will be time to assess how things are going. So – remember that list of statements you rated at the start of the chapter? Well, read and rate them again (I've listed them below, so that you don't have to flick back).

Please score the following questions for breathing on a scale of 1 to 10, with 1 being "not at all true for me" and 10 being "completely true for me".

- When I take a regular breath, my tummy pushes out before my chest.
- When I hit an obstacle in my day, I pause and take a deep breath before responding.
- I make a conscious effort to use my breath as a focus for calming meditation or me-time everyday.
- I have never had a panic attack or a feeling of tightness in my chest and lack of breath when I'm stressed.
- I am able to exercise for 30 minutes at 60 percent effort without getting out of breath.

Your ultimate aim in terms of a score is 40 or above out of 50 – an 80 percent plus result that shows you have this secret nailed and are really using it to help you live forever young. Keep pushing yourself, however, and do what you can to avoid being complacent and slipping back into bad habits.

If you're implementing the takeaways and practising your chosen action points/techniques, I hope you'll see that your score has improved since the first time you did it. If so, you're well on your way to living more "forever young"! So how's that for a breath of fresh air?

If you're not quite where you want to be, return to the "Over to you" section in order to revisit your key action points and ensure that they still feel relevant to you (see page xx for more advice on revisiting and reassessing your goals).

After you have been practising your new "Breathe" techniques for a while, don't forget to revisit your life-balance wheel at some stage (see page xxii) to keep track of progress in terms of how you feel in this area of your life. This will help you to acknowledge your achievements and to keep making further progress. The more you shade in every segment, the bigger the steps you are making along your path of living forever young!

SECRET 2: MOVE

When we looked at breathing, we touched very lightly on how breathing and exercise work together to improve your lung function. Fun movement – whether weight-training, playing basketball, dancing, yoga, pilates or simply a daily walk, etc. – is the next secret to a longer, healthier, more youthful life. But what's the secret about this, I hear you ask. Well, it's the fact that I'm not talking about fitness. Being fit is great, but this is not the primary aim here. What you really want to achieve is a foundation of all-round health, which is a very different thing, and build your fitness on top of that. Fitness alone is not enough to keep you young – it's no good having a six-pack if your head is in the wrong place and your body is toxic. You need the whole package – as explained in the ten secrets in this book – to really thrive, but moving and exercising is a key component. Being forever young is to feel alive, vibrant, happy and balanced every day – and that's what moving is all about.

In this chapter we'll look at some of the most accessible forms of movement – forms that are available to all of us, no matter how time-pressured our lives. My philosophy is that everyday life presents myriad opportunities for us to get up and move – we've just got too used to sitting down. This chapter is going to show you the secret of how to move in fun ways to get your body strong, flexible and balanced. And don't forget that this will do wonders for clearing and balancing your mind, too, so you generally start feeling better on a daily basis.

But, before you begin, let's look at where you are with your movement right now.

WHERE ARE YOU NOW? (PART 1)

Please score the following questions for moving on a scale of 1 to 10, with 1 being "not at all true for me" and 10 being "completely true for me". Note down your score. Then when you've completed this chapter and implemented its advice, try the questions again.

- If my work is desk-based, I ensure that I get up and move away from my desk at least once an hour throughout my working day.
- I make time for formal fitness at least four times a week, for at least 45 minutes each time.
- I am adventurous about how I keep fit and vary my fitness activities throughout the year – fitness isn't just something that happens at an aerobics class or by pounding the streets on a run.
- I seek out activities that push me physically.
- I rarely feel lethargic – when I'm tired it's a healthy, physical tiredness rather than inertia.

THE NEED FOR MOVEMENT

This is not intended to be a book about how to get fit or exercise. However, I do want to emphasize the benefits of exercise for your short- and long-term health and well-being, and therefore for your longevity.

We know that decreasing the amount of activity – including workout load – that you do weakens the body. So, it stands to reason that if you increase the workload on your body *in the correct way* you strengthen it. This doesn't necessarily mean pumping iron to give you muscles worthy of *The Terminator* or running marathons. This is an important point because although I believe fitness is good for you, I firmly believe it should be fun, too – it's about employing whatever type of movement makes you feel good and alive. Even small changes can improve your circulation, which in turn improves the transportation of oxygen and nutrients to all the cells in your magnificent body. And, don't forget that it's not just your physical body that benefits – with better-nourished cells in your brain, your mind and spirit benefit, too.

According to a study published in the American Heart Association journal *Stroke* in 2013, regular walking (not power-walking – just walking-walking) for an hour a day can cut stroke risk by up to one-third in men aged between 60 and 80 years old, and by two-thirds if you walk up to two hours a day. Other studies show that as little as 20 minutes' gentle exercise, such as walking, every day can significantly reduce the risk of a stroke. These benefits are open to pretty much everyone. Regular exercise also helps to maintain or improve mobility, improve coordination, strengthen bones (which is especially important for women at risk of osteoporosis), detoxify the body, boost immunity and even potentially reduce risk of developing some cancers. In terms of the mind, regular exercise improves concentration, memory and mood. Overall, what's not to love?

> Stay active, exercise, sweat and laugh everyday. You have to move. The body was created to move.
>
> Guru Mukh – Kundalini yoga expert, teacher and author

OLD AND TOOTHLESS ALERT

The late US comedienne Joan Rivers said "I never exercise. If God had meant me to bend over, he would have put diamonds on the floor."

Believe me, everyone can exercise. Regardless of age, size, fitness or disability, everyone can do something. And then they can do something more, and soon start to feel much better for it. One of the most common reasons I hear from people I meet for not exercising is that it's too late – they are too old to start and it will hurt too much. I've heard people say, "I'm getting old, I should slow down." If that sounds like you, please think again. Yes – if you have spent much of your life relatively inactive, the introduction of anything that stretches or works your tendons, sinews, joints and muscles will be uncomfortable at first, and you may ache afterwards. But that doesn't mean that it won't have benefits in the long term. If you slow down, you'll only get older quicker.

Even if you are starting from a completely sedentary lifestyle, with a carefully crafted, gentle development plan, and clear management from an expert, incredibly, you'll notice that your muscles and tendons get stretched out even within a few weeks, and so the aches and pains associated with moving more will lessen. As long as you work gently, pushing only to the limits of your movement but not beyond them, risk of injury will be very low – certainly no greater than for any athlete who might do too much too soon.

In reality, age doesn't have to be the great obstacle that it's often presented as – as long as you build up step by step, and always at the edges of, but within, your comfortable range of motion, that range will improve and you'll start to feel fitter, more flexible, more alive, more energized, more balanced and happier, as well as starting to look better, too.

SECRET 2: MOVE

It's a true story...

There is one person very close to my heart who understands totally how important it is to start small, but to get moving: my sweet and loving mother – or mama, as I call her.

Once upon a time – about five years ago – my mum was living what we might call "the good life". But was it really "good"? She was poisoning her body with the wrong foods and lots of alcohol; she took no exercise. Inevitably, she ended up very overweight, had high cholesterol and low blood pressure, and was on the verge of being diagnosed with Type-II diabetes. Her eyesight was failing and she couldn't walk from one room to another without being in serious pain from arthritis. She was in and out of hospital for various arthritis treatments and operations and was 69 years old.

But conventional medicine wasn't treating the cause – it was trying to fix the symptoms. Her lifestyle, and in particular the amount of time she spent moving her body, needed to change. I took her on one of my retreats, and soon after that she lost 28lb with little effort; it just seemed to fall off her because she stuck to some very simple steps. And why was she able to do this? Because she found it fun. On the retreat she cut out all sugars in her diet and lived on fresh alkaline juices, drinking about five pints a day. She started to feel better immediately. Once she got back from the retreat, she was on a roll: she started using one of my morning yoga DVDs that was only 17 minutes long. She got the taste for feeling better, stronger and more balanced, and was hungry for more. She took the next step, and started swimming most days. She started with just a few lengths and kept building on this, and now she swims about 100 lengths most days – at 74 years of age. At her age swimming was the perfect exercise choice – low impact, aerobic and anaerobic exercise all in one. Once she got her momentum going, she looked and felt so much better and younger, and she decided to get a dog. Now, every day she gets up, gets out in the fresh air and – on top of any formal exercise – takes the dog for a walk.

Most days, she does yoga and goes for a swim. Best of all, she has turned into an adventure queen: now in her mid-70s, she is loving life with a healthy body and with the energy she had when she was a youngster. She has sat at the edge of Victoria Falls, been walking with lions, riding with elephants, and swimming with dolphins. She has made movement a regular part of her life in the most adventurous ways. The way she lives is an inspiration to many people – including me.

All you need to do to make changes, like my mum, is to find a place to start. Whether it's a brisk walk that makes your lungs work harder (a little breathless, but not so that you can't hold a conversation), a hiking holiday with friends, a three-peak challenge for charity, a diving holiday with a dedicated tour operator, or formal resistance and strengthening work in a gym – if it motivates you and gets you moving, it's all good.

YOUNG AND RUTHLESS ALERT

Of course, it's not just my older clients who claim that exercise isn't for them. I have plenty of younger clients who throw out excuses at me about why they don't have time for movement, or can't get into exercise.

All these excuses prompted me to start taking a quick straw poll at my live events around the world: "Hands up if you need to be motivated to exercise regularly." It didn't matter if I took the poll in Malaysia, Singapore, Thailand, Bali, Australia, the Philippines, Spain or the UK – I found that 70 percent of the hands in the audience went up. Yet, if I'm talking in primary schools where the children are between four and ten years old, they look at me with an expression that says, "What are you talking about?" Children love moving – and most will look for any excuse to do it. Well, here's some news: you were once that lively child. All you need to do is reconnect with that inner bounce. If you've forgotten what you loved about moving, here's your homework.

Try it now: Thinking about movement

Think about why children use their bodies so much. I think it's because they aren't trapped in their minds. They naturally seek out what feels good to them and follow their instincts. The only thing that stops us moving like we once could is our mind: as we age, we start to monitor how we move, and restrict it. Moving is natural. Moving is a way back to your younger self, not just physically, but mentally, too.

Jot down at least three ways that you used to love moving and using your body as a child. Perhaps you enjoyed dancing – in a class, a school disco or your living room – or played hopscotch, leapfrog or skipping games. Did you use to love running around the playground playing chase? Or were ball games your thing? Perhaps trampolining, a hula hoop – the list goes on.

When you've made your own list, think about which of these activities might still give you pleasure, and how you might incorporate them into your life. It's dead easy, for example, to find a skipping rope and start using it again. Make a commitment right now to do or book one of these activities this week and, who knows, it might become part of your new exercise regime. How fun is that?

»

One tip: if you can buddy up with someone when doing one of these activities – playing a simple game of catch, for example, or having a game of badminton, with a friend – the benefits you get from the exercise will multiply. The human interaction and often increased coordination required will serve to boost your fitness and feeling of well-being all the more.

EXCUSES, EXCUSES

Which of the following statements ring true for you when it comes to committing to some movement?

- I don't have the time/it takes too long
- I don't like running/the gym/aerobics classes
- I don't have the money
- Yoga is only for really bendy people (or only for girls, or wimps – see below)
- I don't enjoy exercise
- I don't have anyone I can exercise with
- I don't know what to do
- I have too many other things that are more important
- It's too much of an effort
- I don't really see the point of it

These are the most common responses I hear at my events when I'm faced with reluctant movers – and the most common of all is, "I don't have time." Yes, you do. You can make time for it – because it will keep you forever young. Let's try a little exercise (not the movement kind, a self-assessment exercise). Awareness is the first point of any change, so get ready for a positive change after this truth assessment.

- How much time do you spend sitting down each day? Work it out – take yourself through a typical day and work out how many minutes or hours you spend sitting. Write it down.
- Now, write down a list of the activities you do while you sit down (examples: working at a computer, watching TV, talking to clients on the phone, travelling to work, eating, and so on).
- Look at the list. Cross off all the activities that require you to sit down, think about them carefully – eating, working at a desk or using your computer, watching TV, etc. Do you *have* to sit still while you do them? For example, if you're talking to someone on your phone, you could walk and talk; if you're watching TV, you could watch while you hold a yoga pose, or even a plank (you know, that abdominal killer when you're supported on your elbows and toes); if you're driving to work, you could park a few blocks or streets away from the office and walk the rest of the way; or, if you're on the bus or subway, you could get off a stop early. Your body needs to move!

Truth is, life presents us with opportunities for movement – we just don't take them. Why we don't take them is open to debate – it could be pure laziness, but I suspect that it's mostly that we just have got used to sitting and it doesn't occur to us to do things any other way. Little adjustments – walking while talking; stretching while watching; stepping while doing the dishes – are powerful. They support your longevity in such a big way. We have to stop thinking in terms of exercise and start thinking in terms of movement. Frankly, as I said, everyone has time for movement. Here are some of my favourites:

- Set the alarm on your laptop and every 40 minutes get up and do 20–40 jumping jacks (depending on what feels suitable wherever you are). If that is too much for you to start with, or you are less mobile, you can exercise sitting down. If you can pick up a remote you can lift up your arms. Lift them as high up as you can, breathe deeply while doing so, and repeat 10, 20 or 30 times. Just start small and do a little more each day.
- If you work in an office, every hour walk around the office or run up and down the stairs for two minutes. (And, come to think of it, instead of taking the elevator, use the stairs.)
- If you're working at home, twice a day put on some music – turn it up loud – and dance like you mean it. (You can try this in the office, too, if your colleagues are with you, I dare you!)

Watch what happens to your creativity and productivity – after your burst of energy, and upping the heart rate, you will find you are better focused, more inventive and altogether much more productive.

DON'T STOP THERE

So, you've taken my advice, you're moving a bit more in those baby-step ways. Congratulations! Now, time to make it all a bit more formal. Start to look at how to incorporate movement into your daily life in a more focused, "exercise" sense. (Don't panic! We're still taking baby steps.) Remember, once you start to be more *aware* of the importance of integrating as much movement as possible into your life, the *types* of movement – walking, cycling, running, yoga, dancing, t'ai chi or whatever – will start to feel a whole lot more achievable.

Physical training has been an important part of most of my life now. I get a real buzz out of it, and I really feel the difference on the days when I don't work out. I have less mental focus, my productivity goes down and so do my energy levels. I try to do at least one hour of general conditioning and stretching every single day. It might be at the gym, or at home to a DVD, or a yoga class, or swimming, or running or a dance class – it's only one hour out of the 18 I tend to be awake, so I give myself no excuses.

However, I realize that not everyone can spare a given amount of time every day, depending on other commitments. So, do what you can but with the aim of increasing the amount you move every day. You'll find that as you start to make time, time presents itself where once you thought there was none.

Remember: the aim is not to become a professional athlete, but to look and feel younger and to increase your longevity. If you can add more movement, building up to about 40 minutes a day, you'll soon find that you're moving simply because it feels good to you in the short term, and you know it is good for you in the long term.

TYPES OF MOVEMENT

I would need a much bigger book to be able to cover every type of movement available to you. So, for now, I'll look at the main three areas that I practise and teach most often: aerobic exercise, anaerobic exercise and yoga. For each, I'll explain a bit about what it is, how it contributes to living forever young, and give you some examples to help you work that form of movement into your own life. If any of these types of movement appeal to you as much as they do to me, fantastic! But if not, then spend a little time considering what forms of movement do, or could appeal to you more… For example, do you like spending time inside or outside? On your own or with others? Being competitive or not?

Aerobic exercise

In simple terms, aerobic exercise is exercising at an intensity that increases the beating of your heart so that you breathe harder and faster. Oxygen is transported directly to your muscles to keep them moving and you will usually quickly feel out of breath. In effect, oxygen is fuel. Swimming, cycling, running, rebounding (working with a mini trampoline), dancing, playing a sport where you're moving consistently, circuit training, HIIT workouts, stair climbing... these are all forms of aerobic exercise.

Regular aerobic exercise will:

- Strengthen the muscles involved in breathing, improving the airflow in and out of your lungs and the transportation of oxygen around your body.
- Improve your heart's pumping efficiency and reduce your resting heart rate, which prolongs your life; it also lowers high blood pressure.
- Reduce the risk of developing Type-II diabetes, because exercise helps to move glucose (sugar) around your system efficiently, helping to balance out your blood-sugar levels.
- Strengthen muscles and tissues throughout your body, helping you stay stronger for longer.
- Fortify your bones, helping to prevent osteoporosis. Statistically, half of all women will be diagnosed with this disease. Any high-impact aerobic activities (such as jogging, skipping, circuit training, rebounding and so on) can stimulate bone growth and reduce the risk of osteoporosis.
- Boost your red blood cell count, improving the movement of nutrients, including oxygen, around your body.
- Reduce stress and anxiety, and improve mood, again because of increased oxygen intake.
- Improve sleep – making it easier to fall asleep and helping you to sleep more soundly through the night (see page 84

for how this helps you live longer).

- Enhance your posture – when you play sports, your body stops hunching and you move instinctively, strengthening muscles that become tight and taut through excessive sitting.

To help you to increase your own aerobic activity, start an activity diary. Whatever aerobic activity you do each day, log it down. If you are lacking in this form of exercise, find something appropriate to add to your life and make a start – this could be just five minutes of skipping per day, building up gradually, over time. It's much easier to monitor your progress if you have a record of what you've been doing. And monitoring your progress is essential for building up your aerobic power consistently.

It's a true story

To show you how fast things can be turned around, I'd like to share a true story about a client who came to me when she was significantly overweight and suffering from the primary symptoms of MS, including slowly losing her vision, consistent pain, fatigue throughout each day and basic coordination problems – she could hardly walk and was in a lot of pain. After seeing me, she started to consume only raw foods and cut out all of the junk food she'd been eating. She added aerobic training to her daily routine, just within her movement levels and pain threshold. She started off very slowly – literally with a walk from one side of the room to the other – but she monitored what she did with the aim that she would always equal what she had done the day before and if she felt she could go further she would. The walk across the room soon became a walk down her street and eventually evolved into a very light jog. Within just seven months, she had not only achieved a healthy weight, but she had completed her first Olympic-distance triathlon: a continuous 1,500-metre swim, 40-kilometre bike ride, and 10-kilometre run. When I met her, she couldn't have believed that a little bit of aerobic exercise every day could have led her to triathlon success within a year, especially in light of having MS. But that was all it took – step by step, little by little.

Anaerobic exercise

Anaerobic exercise doesn't rely upon oxygen in order to fuel exertion, and it won't make you breathless. Think of it as strength and conditioning – press-ups, squats, dips and weight training are all anaerobic activities. Any pulling exercise that uses your bodyweight as resistance is also anaerobic: rock climbing, or using weight machines, for example. Your own bodyweight is perfect for anaerobic exercise –so you don't need a gym membership!

Here are four examples of bodyweight exercises that you can do at home or even at work in your breaks:

Press-ups x10: Lie on the ground with your hands flat, below your shoulders. Engaging your core and keeping your body in a straight line from shoulders to toes, push up until your arms are fully extended, then gradually bend your arms and lower your body until your chest grazes the floor. Don't rush any of the repetitions, do each one controlled and at a steady pace. For beginners, you can do these on your knees and work up to doing the press-ups with only your toes and hands on the floor.

Holding plank position for 30 seconds to 3 minutes: Lie on the floor, supporting yourself on your elbows and forearms with fingers interlocked. Raise your body up, keeping your toes on the floor and a straight back so your body is one long line from head and shoulders to ankles. Don't hold your breath, take deep controlled breaths throughout this.

Squats x10: From a standing position, with a straight back and your fingers beside your temples, squat down as though you are sitting on the edge of a chair. Keep your knees over your toes and your feet flat on the floor. Stand up again, pushing down through your heels. Breathe deep with each repetition.

Tricep dips x10: Sit on the edge of a desk or other stable surface, with your hands either side of your body, palms flat on the desk and facing forward. Move your body forward and lower yourself towards the floor, keeping your hands on the surface and bending your elbows as you lower yourself down and raise yourself up again.

Do the above sequence of four exercises three times. The aim here is to do this at least once a day because it only takes about 5–10 minutes each time. Think about how often children are moving and how much energy they have. Doing this will ignite something within you by getting you out of your mind and back into activating your body, plus it will bring you more strength and more energy. So set yourself a daily reminder and add it to your schedule. I promise you won't regret it.

Yoga

One of the most powerful forms of exercise I've ever encountered, yoga is good for body, mind and spirit. Learning to move through yoga not only physically sculpts and strengthens the body for prolonged health and youthfulness, it provides a focus for the mind. It's all the elements of living forever young rolled into one.

Fundamentally, yoga strengthens your core muscles – that's all the muscles in your torso and down to your buttocks – and increases your flexibility. And, by the way, you don't have to be bendy to start with. When I went back to gymnastics at about 18 years old, I was very stiff, but I took up yoga and used it as a means to stretch every day. From my very first class I became more flexible and, before long, I was more flexible than I had ever been before. My mother, who took up yoga in her 70s, is now hitting positions that she never achieved in her younger years. She is definitely living forever young – go mama! Think of yoga as a means to warm and lengthen your muscles, just as you can warm and lengthen plasticine in your hands.

I believe that yoga not only strengthens my muscles and mind, but my immune system and spiritual connection, too. I think this is because when I was a gymnast I could show the same levels of physical strength and flexibility I can with yoga, but I was always ill: I was fit, but not healthy. Now, however, I'm rarely ill. Yoga gives me bounce, energy *and* immunity. It gives practitioners a sense of balance and deep calm, naturally releasing tensions and reducing stress levels. As stress is a well-known enemy of your immune system (as well as being a cause of ulcers and high blood pressure), it stands to reason that lessening it through a practice such as yoga will boost your immunity and general health.

In the previous chapter, we looked at how yoga breathing techniques, called *pranayama* (see page 11), can help us to breathe more deeply and fully. But, in fact, yoga is good for just about every system and organ in your body. It will:

- Improve your posture well into old age. The stronger and more flexible you are now the deeper the seeds are sown for your strength, flexibility and balance as you get older. Keep the Zimmer frame at bay!
- Decrease stress levels. Studies show that as little as 12 minutes per day of yoga can reduce levels of the stress hormone cortisol, lower the heart rate and improve mood. Yoga movement relieves your muscles by stretching them out, reduces tension in your body and mind, and deactivates your stress response.
- Encourage blood to flow to your body's vital organs, enriching them with oxygen and nutrients to keep them healthy and therefore functioning efficiently for longer.

34

- Improve feelings of self-control. Yoga teaches us that we can control our mind, rather than the mind controlling us. Learning, then, to let negative or destructive thoughts go during yoga practice, by focusing fully on the movement or posture in hand helps to free the mind from its constant chatter, and to promote an all-pervading sense of being in control of our lives – and our youthfulness – even beyond the moment of practice itself.

- Release muscle pain. Because yoga helps the flow of blood, and therefore the transportation of oxygen and nutrients, into your muscles, it flushes out excess lactic acid – the acid build-up that causes the characteristic stiffness and pain in muscles after a workout (in the short term) and inflexibility (in the long term).

- Improve muscular endurance. Holding poses increases your muscular endurance, making you stronger.

- Improve your sleep. Simple yoga exercises in the evening will help you to shake off the stresses of the day and relax so you can fall asleep more easily and let your body recover as you rest.

Some simple yoga to try

Learn these five simple, starter yoga moves and add them to your routine, daily if you can. They are gentle, relaxing, strengthening, and powerful.

Child's pose (*Shishuasana*)
Sit in a kneeling pose, with your bottom touching your heels and your knees spread apart, lean forward placing your forehead on the ground. Arms can be reaching out »

in front of you or resting back towards your heels. Hold for at least three deep breaths. Relax into this as you stretch your back and calm your nervous system.

Cat stretch (*Marjariasana*)

Give your digestive organs an internal massage, improve your digestion and relax your mind with this pose, which is great for a flexible spine. Get down on all fours, with your hands shoulder-width apart, knees hip-width apart and a straight back. Starting with your head looking down at your hands, tilt your pelvis forward and push your belly down, stretching your back and looking up towards the sky. Slowly come back to your starting position and then arch your back the other way, pulling your belly in and moving your chin towards your chest. Do this two or three times, slowly and deliberately.

Butterfly pose (*Baddha Konasana*)

Remove tiredness from standing or walking for long periods, by stretching out your groin and those inner thighs and knees. Sit on the floor with the soles of your feet touching each other and your heels as close to your groin as is comfortable. Gently stretch your inner thighs and see how close you can get your knees to the floor. Hold for a minute or two, getting a little closer to the floor with each out-breath.

Forward bend (*Hastapadasana*)

Stretches your back and hamstrings while invigorating your system because of the increase in blood supply. Stand with your legs just apart and raise your arms

»

above your head. Then, stretch your arms straight out in front of you and bend forward, with your back straight. Bend right over, keeping your knees slightly bent if you have any knee issues or tight hamstrings, and let your head drop down. Hold onto your ankles if you can and breathe deeply. Bring yourself back up to a standing position slowly and repeat the exercise one or two more times.

Legs up the wall (*Viparita Karani*)

Lie down on your back with your bottom against a wall and your legs at a right angle as flat as possible against the wall, arms stretched out to your sides with palms upwards. With your eyes closed simply take deep relaxed breaths in and out and relax into this pose.

As with other new activities in your life, start small and build up slowly. If you already practise yoga, fantastic! Keep doing what you're doing and aim to extend your practice to a more advanced level. If you are just starting out, practise one or two moves, and some *pranayama* breathing (see page 11) for just a few minutes every day. Join a class or follow an online video or yoga book. As you begin to see the benefits to your health, posture and strength, you may want to increase your practice – I encourage you to! It worked for me, it worked for my mum, it has worked for hundreds of my clients and it can work for you, too! Every town (and even village) these days has a beginner's yoga class. For starting out, practising with a teacher to guide you into the postures correctly is probably the safest and most effective way. My sincere hope is that once you start, you won't want to stop.

MOVEMENT AND BREATHING

In the previous chapter, we looked at how to improve each breath when we are in a resting state. Hopefully, you're now breathing into your diaphragm automatically, every day and with every breath. Here, we're going to look at bringing the two together – breathing well during exercise (and for this bit, we are going to talk about exercise, rather than movement – although obviously the rules apply whatever you're doing), so that you can get a double whammy of benefit in your quest to live forever young.

When you exercise, you want to work your muscles to an optimum level. If you are not breathing well, you will be out of breath well before you break into a sweat. Most experts agree that the best breathing pattern during exercise is to breathe in through your nose and out through your mouth. It creates a regular respiration rate, but doesn't dry out your throat.

Whether you're jogging, dancing, playing sports or working out on a cardio machine, try a two-count pattern for your breathing: breathe in through your nose for two counts and then out through your mouth for two counts. You may need to play around with the counts and vary the rhythm, however, to find a count that is comfortable for you. That's fine – just keep it regular and rhythmic so you find your flow.

Once you have established a good rhythm to fit with the pace of your exercise, you should be able to get the oxygen flow you need to get your body moving in time with the flow of your breath. It should come to feel a bit like being in a trance – a natural, rhythmic and regular pattern that eventually you'll do without even having to think about it. This is what athletes do when they're running, cycling and swimming for long distances. It also helps stop the mind from coming up with thoughts that don't serve you. If it helps, find music to breathe and exercise along to.

Here are some other suggestions to help you get your breath and exercise in rhythm:

- According to breathing expert Alison McConnell, author of *Breathe Strong, Perform Better*, lots of runners aim to have one breath for each two foot strikes. In other words, you breathe in while you take two steps (one right and one left) and two steps while you breathe out. This is known as the 2:2 rhythm, and it's a bit like breathing in and out for a count of two.
- Remember to breathe from your diaphragm (see page 6), as deep breaths will help you to find a long, regular and sustainable rhythm during your exercise, which is more meditative and restorative for your mind as well as your body.
- While you're breathing in through your mouth and out through your nose, try to maintain a bit of a contraction on the back of your throat so that you sound a little like Darth Vader from *Star Wars*. Being able to hear your breath in this way will help you to keep to a rhythm. You'll notice that this is opposite to the breathing technique of in through the nose and out through the mouth that I mentioned earlier. This is simply because when you're exerting yourself with these types of exercises you can inhale more oxygen through your mouth more easily – you will naturally tend to do this.

AIMS – NOT RULES – OF ENGAGEMENT

I'm not necessarily one for strict rules in life because things are changing so fast in today's world that we need to be able adjust fast and be flexible, but when it comes to movement, having a few rules can help you to get into a rhythm of seeing just exactly how easy it can be to bring fun exercise into your life. However, because no one likes rules, let's call them aims.

- Start gently and build up gradually. For example, start with a set time frame for what you're going to do and increase it only when you feel the urge to, don't push yourself unnecessarily because that can lead to a build up of acid, which doesn't help with living forever young. So, if you're at the beginning, it might be a five-minute walk until you get out of breath. Once you can do that comfortably, then, little by little, start adding a few minutes each time to it until you get to about 40 minutes. Once you've reached that, then in the middle of those walks, add a little jog in for about 30 seconds and then walk again until you have your breath back. Increase this over time until you can do the entire 40 minutes jogging. This can apply to any movement that requires aerobic activity, and it will do wonders for getting your heart strong but do this at a pace that you're comfortable with. Don't forget to use the wisdom of baby steps here.
- Get slightly out of breath a few times every day, but don't push it – you should be a little breathless, not speechless.
- Never ignore bad pain – listen to your body because it may be telling you to temporarily stop, before you do some damage. Remember, though, that there is good pain and bad pain – good pain is a stretching pain, and it's really, if you think about it, bearable; bad pain makes you wince and perhaps even shout "Ouch!"
- Never, ever push yourself when you have a bad cold or flu symptoms. If you are feverish, stay on the sidelines, then work up to a short walk when you feel up to it.
- Move with other people – if you make it sociable and fun, you're more likely to move more. And, besides, if you can hold a conversation while moving, you know you're going at the right pace. It's good for the mind and soul, too, to connect with someone else during activity.
- Mix it up with normal life. Try to fit some exercise into your daily routine – stretch out your glutes (butt muscles)

while you sit on the bus (cross an ankle over the opposite knee and press down on the raised knee) and lean slightly forward until you feel the stretch. Walk a bus stop instead of riding the bus; take a skipping rope into your local park in your lunch hour and do a little skipping – even just a few minutes will make a big difference. While you're watching TV, get used to holding a static yoga pose or practise some light stretching. You don't have to stretch for the entire length of a TV show or a film, but a few minutes every hour is a much better use of your time than practising the couch potato pose!

- On days when you have a bit more time, go to a local yoga class or for a jog. And don't forget team sports – find a local club offering Back to Netball, Back to Hockey, or an equivalent, or try a local soccer team. Most sports have sessions that will suit any ability. And, if all else fails, dance round your living room like no one is watching and really give yourself that freedom. I have no doubt that you'll love it.

- Find a mountain and climb it; find a river and paddle it; find a beach and run along the shore; find a sea and swim it; find a forest and ramble through it – get out into nature when you can and turn movement into adventure.

- Persist! Physical activity can offset age-related disease and decline, so don't just read this, implement these gifts into your lifestyle so you actually feel the benefits. It may have taken you years to get out of shape, but just a week or two of even a slow reintroduction will show benefits.

It's a true story...

My family has a tendency to become overweight. It's in our genes, they say. When my nephew hit rock bottom, the biggest and unhealthiest he had ever been, he realized he was really unhappy – with himself and his life. He had no focus, and he didn't like the way he looked. He was 24 years old.

I persuaded him to start coming to the gym with me. In the early days, he wasn't lifting heavy weights, but he was making an effort – both in being there, and gradually in the exercises he was doing. Together, we celebrated every set, every session. He was doing something that felt good and he was getting better at it. Before long, he developed confidence, his mood swings abated, his body shape changed. Progress was slow and steady, but sustainable. Now he is no longer overweight and has completely turned around his life. Initially through movement and exercise, he has realized his own greatness – a greatness that he'll take with him throughout his life's journey. He has a new job, which he feels his newfound energy and confidence helped him get, and is happy, healthy and strong. He has combined his increase in movement with dietary changes and a development of his self-belief – he is a living embodiment of my ten secrets for living forever young and his enjoyment of life is truly infectious.

ENJOY IT

I want to finish this chapter with one essential message, even though we've already mentioned it earlier: however you move, make sure you enjoy it. Not only does increased movement play a great role in balancing out hormones, I believe it gives more space for your spirit to breathe through you. It would be really hard to live forever young without living in the joy of movement.

Joan Rivers (who lent us her words of wisdom at the start of the chapter) also said, "The first time I see a jogger smiling I'll try it." And she's right. There's no point in punishing yourself. If you hate jogging, try something else. If you tire of the something else, find another something else again – when you think in terms of the adventure of movement, the possibilities are endless. Walking, cycling, swimming, dancing, climbing, caving, rowing… whatever gets you moving *and* makes you feel happy is right for you. Even though moving releases happy hormones, movement will only really lift your spirit if you enjoy it in the first place.

NOW YOU CAN MOVE

Movement is more than exercise – it is a connection with your body in a way that makes you feel good. I hope you've come to realize in this chapter not just how important exercise is for your body, but how it must also be fun in order to nourish your mind and spirit. That means that movement doesn't have to be formal, and that you are never too old or too young, and you never have too little time. Movement is for everyone.

LIVING FOREVER YOUNG
TOP 10 TAKEAWAYS: MOVE

- Find time for movement – even if it's a walk in your lunch hour or some exercises in the staff room. Get moving!
- Watch children at play – see how they move without inhibition. Try to recapture some of that freedom in your own movement.
- Be confident about your ability to move – go to the edge of your comfort zone, but take baby steps to get there.
- Make movement fun! If you hate running, don't do it! Find something else instead. If lifting weights would be like lifting lead to you, find other ways to get active.
- Use the need to move as a trigger for adventure – that way it nourishes your spirit as well as your body and mind.

- Try some resistance training at home – using your own bodyweight. A few tricep lifts against the sofa while you're watching TV sounds like a great use of time to me!
- Reduce the stress in your mind by getting back into your body – while you're focusing on your movement, there's less time for your mind to be distracted by stress.
- Use movement as a means to breathe more air – get outside and do it, get your heart pumping and your lungs moving. That's two secrets for the price of one!
- Use your movement choices as a way to connect with others – group classes or walking with friends means time when you're connecting in a shared experience or adventure.
- Daily movement brings together all these elements for the good of your mind, body and spirit. What are you waiting for?!

OVER TO YOU

Now that you've read the bulk of this chapter, it's time for you to choose how exactly you are going to make the secrets of good moving *your own* by integrating them into your daily life. So…

- Close the book and consider the ways in which you would feel most able and happy to start putting this chapter's suggestions, or any other moving-related ideas of your own that you have, into practice.
- Then take a pen and notebook or piece of paper and write down the three, or five, of these ways that you most like the idea of really committing to, and that you feel will not only be really useful for you, but also achievable and sustainable. For example, you might decide to set an alarm every hour while you're at work and do something fun to move your body for 1–3 minutes; choose a regular time

in your week to ensure that you get out into the great outdoors to move your body, whether walking, running, cycling, climbing or whatever else; and/or find a friend or neighbour to diary in some fun activities with so that you're accountable to one another and therefore all the more likely to stick to your plans.

- If the thought of three or five things overwhelms you, just start with one – baby steps are the best way to go and as long as you keep up what you have started you'll soon find momentum building and you will want to, and be able to, do more.

- If you need a little help and encouragement to get into this decision-making zone, try the "Lost in Music" technique on page xxi to set you on your way.

- Then read your chosen action points out loud to yourself – and make an inward commitment about how, when and where you're going to start putting them into practice – as of this week, or even *today* if possible. Feel free to write these practical details beneath the action points if you feel it will help you stick at them...

- Now use this list as your personal guide to enhancing the "Move" section of your life-balance wheel, coming back to the list any time you feel the need to revise it or add to it...

WHERE ARE YOU NOW? (PART 2)

Once you have been using the above list of action points for about a month, it will be time to assess how things are going. So – remember that list of statements you rated at the start of the chapter? Well, read and rate them again (I've listed them below, so that you don't have to flick back).

Please score the following questions for moving on a scale of 1 to 10, with 1 being "not at all true for me" and 10 being "completely true for me".

- If my work is desk-based, I ensure that I get up and move away from my desk at least once an hour throughout my working day.
- I make time for formal fitness at least four times a week, for at least 45 minutes each time.
- I am adventurous about how I keep fit and vary my fitness activities throughout the year – fitness isn't just something that happens at an aerobics class or by pounding the streets on a run.
- I seek out activities that push me physically.
- I rarely feel lethargic – when I'm tired it's healthy, physical tiredness rather than inertia.

Your ultimate aim in terms of a score is 40 or above – an 80 percent plus result that shows you have this secret nailed and are really using it to help you live forever young. Keep pushing yourself, however, and do what you can to avoid being complacent and slipping back into bad habits.

If you're implementing the takeaways and practising your chosen action points/techniques, I hope you'll see that your score has improved since the first time you did it. If you're not quite where you want to be, return to the "Over to you" section in order to revisit your key action points and ensure that they still feel relevant to you (see page xx for more advice on revisiting and reassessing your goals).

After you have been practising your new "Move" techniques for a while, why not revisit your life-balance wheel (see page xxii) to keep track of progress and see how things have changed in terms of how you feel in this area of your life. This will help you to acknowledge your achievements and to keep making further progress. The more you shade in every segment, the bigger the steps you are making along your path of living forever young!

SECRET 3: NOURISH

It goes without saying that your body needs nourishment
to survive. However, living forever young is not just about
surviving, it's about thriving. Your body takes the goodness –
the vitamins, minerals, healthy fats and other nutrients – out
of the food you eat and turns it into energy to fuel your body
and mind. The leftovers become waste, which your body then
eliminates. This entire process is what we call your digestion,
and we need your digestion to be healthy in order for you to
be properly nourished in a way that helps to keep all your body
systems functioning efficiently.

When your diet falls short (and it happens to the best of
us), a good-quality supplement regime can step in to fill the
gaps but remember, supplements are just that – supplement
to a healthy diet, not a replacement for it... more of that later.
And then there's water – the life-giving hydration that is so
fundamental to the health of your body's cells, and a metaphor
for a fluidity that enables you to get the most out of your life.

In this chapter we'll look at the secrets of good nutrition
– how you can optimize your diet through the correct foods
that you eat and the dietary principles you can follow, and the
role that the right type of nutritional supplements can play in
making sure your body has everything it needs so you can be
living forever young. Then we'll look deeper into water – or
more specifically at hydration for your body and mind – and
consider how water is fundamental to a healthy life and a
healthy spirit.

But, before we begin, let's look at where you are with your
nourishment right now.

WHERE ARE YOU NOW? (PART 1)

Please score the following questions for nourishment on a scale of 1 to 10, with 1 being "not at all true for me" and 10 being "completely true for me". Note down your score. Then, when you've completed this chapter and implemented its advice, try the questions again.

- I am aware of my diet and try to eat healthily every day.
- I look forward to preparing and make all my main meals from scratch.
- I eat foods that sustain my energy levels all day, rather than relying on caffeine or sugar.
- I take combined, natural supplements and superfoods only as a safeguard to fill any gaps in my healthy diet.
- I make sure that I drink at least two litres of quality alkaline water a day, more when I exercise.

THE NEED TO NOURISH

In the developed world, by and large, we mostly eat too much of the wrong stuff. I'm talking about processed foods, foods that now have harmful chemicals in them, foods that have had essential fats removed to be replaced with sugars and sweeteners, and foods filled with harmful salts. If you put junk food into your body, your body will start to feel like junk. It really is that simple.

If, on the other hand, you put fresh, nutrient-rich, pesticide-free food into your body, you will feed it the purest nutrients firing off the best-quality energy. You'll strengthen your immune system, feel and look more healthy (and more youthful), and even help to prolong your life. Again, it's simple.

YOU ARE WHAT YOU EAT

So, what do I mean by junk food? I'm not just talking about the
meals served up by your local fast-food joint. Junk food presents
itself in many ways. Take foods laden with preservatives, for
example. Up until about 100 years ago, the methods available
for preserving foods were wholly natural: salting, pickling,
smoking, drying, fermenting and so on. These natural methods
of preserving food and its nutrients enabled our ancestors to
enjoy a nutrient-rich diet even when fresh food was scarce at
certain times of year.

Over time, food manufacturers began using artificial
preservatives to prolong shelf life – this made seasonal and non-
indigenous foods more widely available throughout the year
and across continents. While that gives us a wonderful degree
of choice, it also means we are at risk of ingesting manmade
chemicals that your body is not designed to tolerate. Similarly,
the use of artificial pesticides and herbicides to preserve crops
while they are in the soil increases our exposure to more
manmade chemicals.

In addition, while fast foods seem to be packed with
flavour, in fact this is often largely as a result of the lavish use
of "bad" oils (saturated fats), and harmful processed salts or
refined sugars. Some studies, including one published in the
British Journal of Sports Medicine in 2017, claim that sugar
is addictive, like some recreational drugs. Although that
claim received a backlash from other members of the medical
profession, it is generally accepted that, rather like the use of
table salt, using sugar is at the very least habitual – once you
get used to the taste of it, you can't remember what food or
drink tasted like without it.

Processed foods that contain high levels of salt, sugar or fat
– or a combination of any of these – often have also had most of
their natural goodness removed and contain significant numbers

of artificial additives, making them nutritionally depleted. As a result they don't have a place in the diet of someone who wants to live forever young. Instead, I want to encourage you to eat foods that are closer to their natural state – that means seasonal, organic foods, and as many raw fruits and vegetables as possible.

EAT ORGANIC

Grown or farmed without any chemical pesticides, fungicides, herbicides, steroids, growth hormones or preservatives, organic foods come from chemical-free soils – soils that must also be chemical-free for miles around. However, it's worth noting that the specific regulations about which foods can be certified organic can vary from country to country, so do check the regulations for your region and buy your food accordingly.

If your budget doesn't stretch to a full organic diet, make organic choices for key ingredients. For example, choose organic meat and fish, but buy non-organic vegetables, just making sure you wash and peel them as appropriate. Although non-organic veg can have chemicals from the soil in the flesh of the food itself, you can at least remove the surface bad guys. Many supermarkets also now sell food wash, specifically formulated (from natural ingredients) to remove chemical residue from the surface of foods.

EAT FRESH AND WHOLE

Fruit and vegetables lose significant amounts of vitamins and minerals in the "short" period of time between harvesting and reaching your table. The best way to eat fresh and whole fruit and vegetables is to find local farmers and producers, and buy directly from source. If you aren't able to get to a local farm shop or you don't have one nearby where you can buy your foods as soon as they are harvested, your best bet may be to buy foods that were frozen immediately upon being gathered or picked.

A "whole food" is food that arrives at your table exactly as Mother Earth intended – with all its nutrients intact, and free from additives and other artificial substances. Whole foods, by definition, contain all the correct balance of nutrients and micronutrients to make them nutritionally "perfect" for your body. Think of it like food synergy – perfect togetherness – that nourishes your body, creating synergy in your own body systems, too.

Whole foods are not only whole fresh fruit and vegetables, but whole grains, too – and foods such as brown pasta and rice, which are made using the whole grain, unprocessed, rather than the stripped-back white version that has had a lot of its nutrients removed. They are picked in season, when the plants are ripe, and naturally provide the best nutrients for your body. A diet rich in whole, fresh, organic produce will make you feel so much more alive than one heavy in processed, chemical-laden food.

EAT MORE PLANTS

No, not the ones in the garden (unless you're growing your own fruit, veg and herbs, of course). Try to modify your diet to eat more plant-based foods, which are rich in diverse nutrients and have been linked to lower rates of chronic illness, rather than meat or fish. I live on mostly plant-powered foods so I'm vegan but I'm not suggesting that you *have* to become vegetarian or vegan, unless of course you want to. I'm simply suggesting that you reduce the amount of meat in your diet (see page 61). Even if you have only a couple of meatless days per week, you will notice a difference in your bowel movements (you'll be clearing waste from your body more effectively) and increased

energy levels – because all the energy your body uses struggling
to digest meat is diverted into pure, unadulterated zeal for life!
At my total immersion courses (total immersion means we all
stay together day and night, and have all our meals supplied),
we provide only plant-based foods. Although, at the start of
the course, some participants may be resistant to the notion of
giving up meat and dairy, within a few meals, when energy levels
start to soar and people feel and look better and healthier, any
barriers that existed start to break down. Many people go on
to continue eating a plant-strong diet as a lifestyle choice when
they get back to the "real world".

I believe that plant-based foods, or plant-powered foods
as I like to call them, are brilliant at helping you to live longer.
There are lots of reasons why, so here are just a few to whet
your appetite:

- Plant foods contain antioxidants, which help your body
  to neutralize free radicals, the unstable atoms that cause
  ageing and even contribute to certain diseases such as cancer
  and heart disease. Plants of similar colours contain similar
  antioxidants, so eating a rainbow of fruit and vegetables
  ensures your body is receiving a vibrant cocktail of benefits.
- Green leafy vegetables, such as spinach and kale, contain
  good amounts of vitamin K, which can help the body stave
  off age-related diseases such as osteoporosis (bone-wasting)
  and heart disease.
- Aubergines contain a compound called nasunin, a potent
  antioxidant that can protect the nerve cells in your brain,
  potentially prolonging mental acuity.
- Fruit and vegetables high in vitamin C help to prevent
  skin-ageing because vitamin C is believed to boost
  collagen production – the compound that gives your
  skin its elasticity.
- Brassica vegetables (such as Brussels sprouts, cabbage and

cauliflower) and those from the allium family (garlic and onions primarily) contain sulphur compounds that can help to ease the pain of inflammation in bones and joints – a key cause of pain in age-related arthritis.

- The Nuffield Department of Clinical Medicine at the University of Oxford released research in 2011 showing that vegans and vegetarians present a decreased risk of developing cataracts compared to meat eaters.

- A vegan or vegetarian diet carries a proven reduced risk of developing age-related (Type-II) diabetes – the George Washington University School of Medicine has stated that, "vegetarian diets offer an important benefit for the management of diabetes and can even reduce the likelihood of development by one half." Cool stuff!

Another reason, albeit controversial and still being studied, could be that a plant-based diet can help to preserve the "length" of the little bits of DNA that sit at the ends of your chromosomes, called telomeres. One scientist has described these like the little bits of plastic wrapping that you get at the ends of shoelaces. These wear away as you age – but that wear and tear is hastened through poor dietary choices. If you follow good dietary principles, and pack your diet full of whole foods and fresh fruits and vegetables, some scientists believe you can slow down and reverse the speed of this wear and tear, prolonging cell life.

Overall, evidence suggests that widespread adoption of a vegetarian diet could prevent approximately 40,000 deaths in Great Britain alone each year – that's a lot of people living longer!

Vegetable-based diet and whole nutrition

If you're of the opinion that all vegans and vegetarians have nutritional deficiencies, please think again. The official position of the American Dietetic Association is that "a comprehensive and well-designed vegetarian, or vegan, diet can be nutritionally sound and appropriate for all ages and stages of life, including infants, the elderly, and even athletes. Being healthy can reduce incidences of disease, and better management of existing health problems are all associated with following a vegetarian diet." Basically, as long as you eat a broad range of beans, pulses, seeds, nuts, veg and fruit, you can get all the nutrition you need from a vegetarian or vegan diet.

EAT RAW

In my view, it's not just vegetables that need upping in a diet in the quest to live forever young, but also the amount of vegetables we eat raw. Raw foods come to you exactly as nature intended: without any of the nutritional depletion that occurs during cooking.

The easiest way to increase the amount of raw veggies in your diet is to have a raw vegetable-based juice or smoothie every day. A word of advice: buy yourself a good juicer for your juices and a good blender for your smoothies – the best you can afford. Making your own juices and smoothies is super easy if you have a piece of kit that does the job efficiently, and is easy to clean! And if you make them yourself, then you have the added bonus of knowing exactly what's gone into what you're drinking!

Fresh juices and smoothies are rich in live enzymes, which are essential for the efficient running of your digestive system and provide catalysts for the function of and communication between all the cells in your body. In fact, enzymes are essential for most of the building and rebuilding that goes on in the body every day. Cooking destroys these precious enzymes, which is why raw foods are so important.

I like to have a green vegetable-based juice pretty much first thing every morning, before I eat breakfast (see opposite).

Three of my favourite drinks

Morning Green Juice
Play around with different combinations and amounts
of the below ingredients until you find a mix you love:

> Kale
> Celery
> Cucumber
> Apple
> Spinach
> Lemon
> Ginger

Superfood Berry Smoothie
Again, play with different combinations and amounts
of the below ingredients to taste. Any of the fruits
can be kept frozen for ease. Go easy with the amount
of superfoods you add at first as some of them can
have quite a strong flavour; then up the amount as
you grow to love their positive effects!

> Strawberries
> Blueberries
> Blackberries
> Goji berries
> Mulberries
> Water, nut milk or coconut milk
> A mix of superfoods: wheatgrass, barley grass,
>   chlorella, spirulina and hemp protein

»

Tropical Smoothie
Below is another combination to try. Adding a couple of spoonfuls of linseeds, flaxseeds or hemp seeds to this smoothie really makes it pack a punch!

Banana
Blueberries
Coconut milk
2 scoops of your favourite nuts or seeds

I often follow this up mid-morning with a superfood berry smoothie (see page 57) because while a freshly squeezed juice will fast-track nutrients straight into your bloodstream, a smoothie (which includes the whole fruit) will provide the added benefit of using the flesh of the vegetables and fruit, giving you the fibre, too. It's good for your digestion and will stop you reaching for that sugary snack. Smoothies are also great vehicles for superfoods – such as wheatgrass, barley grass, chlorella, spirulina, hemp protein, chia, cacao, the list goes on – to further boost your nutritional intake.

Another tip on how to get more raw veggies into your diet is to eat a raw salad (including some grated or shredded vegetables, as well as leaves) before or with your main meal every day. Something as simple as a bowl of leaves topped with grated carrot, sliced beetroot or courgette and drizzled with a balsamic vinaigrette, with some fresh lemon and extra virgin olive oil is a quick, easy and, above all, tasty addition to your daily diet that will help you on your way to living forever young – feeling more energized and looking great.

EAT ALKALINE

The natural pH (potential Hydrogen) of our blood is slightly alkaline, usually between a pH of 7.35 and 7.45. In simplest terms, the higher the pH reading, the more alkaline and oxygen-rich you are; the lower the pH reading, the more acidic and oxygen-deprived you are. An acidic body provides an environment in which disease, including age-related diseases such as heart issues and certain cancers, can thrive and which accelerates cell ageing.

The foods that you eat affect your body's pH levels. Slightly acidic foods, such as beans and nuts, eaten in moderation are not harmful to you; but those that are extremely acidic, such as meat, processed foods, refined white foods and alcohol, can negatively affect your health. On the other hand, highly alkaline foods will help to ensure that your body is working at optimum efficiency. Alkalising foods include most fruits and vegetables (dark green leafy veg and sea vegetables, such as the various types of edible seaweed are particular superstars) as well as herbs, spices and flower teas, such as dandelion tea.

FOODS TO KEEP OFF THE MENU

Inevitably, if some foods are good for you, some are not. The following are the foods that I advise you to reduce or remove entirely from your diet in your quest to live forever young, in addition to the processed foods that have already been mentioned.

"Low" foods

Low-cal, low-fat, low-sugar… Don't be tempted to believe that these labels mean the contents of the packet are good for you. Most "low" foods have had something natural removed, or even if they are replacing something unnatural and "bad" for you (such as refined sugar), the chances are that it's a straight swap with something equally bad, if not worse, which is usually a manmade chemical.

What is more, while low-fat yogurts may have fewer calories, many nutritional studies show that eating moderate amounts of natural fats (that is, fats found in food naturally, not those added to food to make them taste better) have the effect of improving overall balance in the diet and reducing incidence of obesity. In addition, low-fat and low-calorie foods often have added sugar to make them more palatable. And added sugar is definitely a no-no. Overall then, steer clear.

Sugary foods

Research shows that when sugar enters the body, it reacts with certain proteins and hardens the collagen (connective tissue) in your skin. The tangible result of that is that it accelerates skin-ageing, causing dry patches and wrinkles. Furthermore, sugar itself provides empty calories – it is of no nutritional benefit to your body at all.

If you have a sweet tooth and feel that you can't get by without sugar, try at first to simply steer clear of *refined white sugar*, in all its forms. While it's okay to replace it with a little natural sugar – such as coconut sugar, maple sugar, honey or agave nectar – while you get used to less sugary tastes, bear in mind that sugar is sugar. It is never healthy. Ever. So switch to natural forms, but then start to reduce the amount you use in your cooking and wean yourself off adding it to drinks, such as tea and coffee, and cereals.

You may wonder about sugar naturally found in fruits. Adding or using extracted fruit sugar as a refined sugar replacement is no better for you than using refined sugar in the first place. However, eating a moderate amount of whole fruits, including the sugar that they contain, is fine – the fibre in the fruit flesh helps to balance out the effects of the fruit sugar in your body. Just make sure you don't eat fruit in excess and be sure to look after your teeth as the effect of fruit sugar directly on the pearly whites is barely any better than boiled sweets.

Fortified foods

A note on fortified foods: these are foods, most often breakfast cereals, that loudly proclaim the fact that they include (are "fortified with") additional vitamins. Merely adding vitamins into food through fortification does not give the same nutritional value as those vitamins in the same quantities in fresh foods or in a good-quality supplement. Get your nutrients in ways that are raw, unprocessed and integral (more of that later).

Meat and fish

I am not expecting every reader of this book to become vegetarian, and I accept that meat-eating is still a perfectly normal part of most people's lives. However, the concentrated protein in meat makes it very difficult for your body to digest – some meats can sit in your gut for three days before your body has effectively broken them down before elimination. Furthermore, one study by the University of Glasgow, UK, published in 2016, found links between the consumption of red meat as part of an overall poor diet and increased signs of ageing, particularly in the kidneys.

So if you like the idea of a meat-free diet, be assured that you can get all the protein you need from a varied diet that includes plenty of fruit, vegetables, nuts, beans, pulses, seeds and grains.

However, if you would still prefer to eat at least some meat, follow these rules to minimize the negative effects on your health:

- Limit meals of fish or meat to only two or three times a week.
- Opt for white meat or fish over red meat.
- Choose organic meat (before you choose organic fruit and vegetables, if you have to make a choice).
- Choose fish that is rich in healthy omega-3 and omega-6 fatty acids, which the body can't manufacture for itself and we have to derive from our food – salmon, mackerel, sardine and herring are good examples of this.
- However, avoid eating oily fish, such as tuna, salmon, marlin and swordfish, more than twice a week – this is because oily fish can contain high levels of mercury, a harmful toxin.
- Avoid eating carbs and meat together – the body breaks down carbohydrate foods, such as potatoes, rice and wholegrain pasta, faster than it breaks down meat, so it's easier on your digestion if you eat them separately.

Dairy products

As a child I had any number of allergies, very bad skin conditions and many breathing ailments. I have traced most of them back to dairy products – milk, cheese, yoghurt... Of course, not everyone will react to dairy foods the way I did (or do). However, there is much controversy about whether or not dairy is as good for us as we once thought. Some researchers claim that the body uses up more calcium than it gains in the breakdown of dairy plus it contains lactic acid which your body must buffer from your bones and organs, while others maintain that dairy has only nutritional benefit for the body and that it is essential for the health of the bones.

I am vegan, so I eat no dairy products at all, replacing cow's milk with alternatives such as coconut milk, almond milk, cashew nut milk, rice milk and, if I can't source those, then rarely I'll use soya milk. I make sure I get good amounts of calcium by packing my diet full of dark leafy green vegetables, figs and almonds, which are all great sources. And I feel so much better for it. If, however, giving up dairy is not for you, just make sure that the dairy products you do eat are from organic farms and grass-fed animals.

Diet and dieting

No one who eats a healthy array of nutritionally balanced foods should need to "diet" as such, that is restrict food intake for the purposes of losing weight. A healthy attitude to food means that you will settle at your optimum weight, shape and look and feel absolutely fabulous for the rest of your life.

However, many experts believe that you should eat according to your age, to optimize your health at each stage in your life. Let me explain… if you look at animals in nature they aren't overweight and never need to count calories. When selecting fresh, plant-powered foods, your body gets in tune with your life and when it is satisfied with the amount of food it needs, it fires a signal to your brain to stop you eating and over-indulging. Eat well and listen to your body and you will settle at your right weight. The amount of food you need depends on your age and your lifestyle – a physically demanding job requires more calories than sitting at a desk for most of the day, for example – and no one knows your body like you do, because you live in it. Make sure that the food you eat is for nutritional, not emotional, purposes and you'll soon be in balance with your choices and know when you've had enough. Let your body do the talking and pay attention to it.

YOUR DIET: STARTING OVER

If you've been reading all this and feeling that you need to make some changes in order to eat better and feel better, don't panic. You don't need to do everything overnight. Give yourself time to adjust, introducing new dietary principles little by little, until they become natural and habitual. Change at your own pace, and get used to one or two healthier alternatives before tackling more. This way, you're more likely to stick with the healthy changes that you make. So, for example, during the first two weeks of your new, youthful diet, you might simply introduce a veggie-based juice or smoothie before breakfast three mornings a week, increasing to every day after this. In week four, you might then replace one meat-based meal with a veggie one – increasing week on week, until you have hit a balance that makes you feel at your best. Or, one week you might switch that packet of crisps you have every day to a handful of raw almonds and walnuts. (They are tasty and crunchy, not to mention nutritious and unprocessed.) The following week, you might switch your mid-morning doughnut for a fruit salad, or some healthy crackers, spread with a little nut butter or hummus. And so on. The key, as with everything, is to take a little time to really think about what is likely to work for you because the idea appeals to you and you believe you'll feel better for it. Otherwise, you're unlikely to be able to sustain your new "youthful" eating habits.

Kick-start with a juice cleanse

The world today is more toxic than ever with pollution and pesticides affecting our environment and our food. I believe that we need to detox and cleanse our bodies on a regular basis. A two- or three-day juice cleanse (see overleaf) will give your body a chance to reboot, rest and recover – it helps your system to catch up with the housekeeping that it needs to do to keep it working optimally. I recommend doing this at least four times a year, as the seasons change, but if you have any medical issues whatsoever you should check with your doctor first.

Juice cleanse

Simply start your day with a glass of warm water flavoured with a squeeze of fresh lemon and then drink 2–2.5 litres of freshly made juice throughout the day and have no other food. I'd suggest breaking this down into five or six drinks, taken at regular intervals, and take your juice ingredients from all the colours of the rainbow. Start with a green juice (such as the one on page 57), so you boost your alkalinity from the word go, then mix and change throughout the day. Some people like a veg-only juice followed by a fruit-only one, so it's rather like having vegetable soup followed by a pudding at each meal time. And really savour each one ...

Don't sweat the small stuff

Food should be fun – and it definitely shouldn't be about denial. You need a balance that makes you feel good. Aim for a ratio of 80:20 – that is, following forever young dietary principles for 80 percent of the time, and allowing yourself indiscretions 20 percent of the time. If you find yourself knee deep in chocolate cake one afternoon, enjoy it and don't feel guilty about it! (Just don't make a habit of it.)

Keep it regular

Eat healthily little and often so that you don't feel hungry – hunger will send you reaching for a sugary quick-fix. And if you feel emotional or tired, don't reach for the confectionary chocolate (you can make the odd exception for raw or dark chocolate of at least 70 percent cacao, not cocoa). Instead, have a soothing cup of raspberry-leaf tea, or a bowl of miso or vegetable soup. Tomato and basil, Thai green curry, carrot and coriander and pumpkin are my favourite comfort-food, veggie soups, and chopped carrots, celery or cucumber dipped in hummus is my go-to tasty and satisfying snack.

Take your time

How many times do you eat on the move, or rush through a meal so that you can get on with another job or watch something on TV or leave to get somewhere? Eating is fundamental to your physical and mental well-being and taking time over your food – eating mindfully and engaging all your senses – is known to be beneficial for your digestion. This is common sense really, we all know that rushing food is bad for you – you can take in too many calories before you realize you have eaten enough, and it leads to indigestion. The optimum way to eat for your body, and your mind, to enjoy food is to take small mouthfuls, making sure you savour the flavours and textures of what you're eating, and take time to chew. Chewing is especially important as it ramps up the digestive process, signalling to your stomach that food is on its way.

Even before you start eating, take some time over the preparation of your food – this again gets your stomach juices whirring and prepares your digestive system for receiving food and breaking it down efficiently. Mindful cooking and eating is, quite simply, kinder to your digestive system.

Say thanks

At my advanced trainings we say a blessing before we eat. This can be a little weird for some people, but the practice of "giving thanks" for food dates back thousands of years. There's no need to think of it in a religious or spiritual sense (unless you want to), but simply as a means to calm your nervous system, reduce any stress and plug into a state in which your body can accept the food's goodness and its ability to nourish you not only physically, but emotionally and mentally, too.

The blessing doesn't need to be complicated, all you need to do is to give thanks. You can simply sit still for a moment and say to yourself or out loud, *Thank you for this food that is about to nourish my body and help me live forever young.*

Alternatively, you can use the following idea, adapting it in any way that feels comfortable to you.

- Set the table and make it look inviting – remember that eating should be a joyful pleasurable experience that engages all the senses.
- Place your food on the table and sit down ready to eat. Place your hands above your food – holding your palms downward. The aim is to sense energy coming from your food and in through energy centres in the palms of your hands.
- Say a few words of thanks, for example: *Thank you to the sun for shining on our planet and helping to feed the plants with your energy. Thank you to the rain that watered this food and helped it to grow. Thank you to the farmers that helped to harvest this food and thank you to the people who made it possible to bring it from the field to my table. Thank you to the person who prepared this meal for me.*

For me, a little exercise like this before I eat or drink anything, even if I just run through it in my head, is as valuable as warming up my body before exercise.

Reconnect

Use mealtimes as opportunities to reconnect with those you love. Sit together as often as you can to discuss the events of the day – make sure that everyone gets a turn to share. Avoid all distraction: no TV, no smartphones, no tablets – make your mealtimes about human interaction and love of each other. Interestingly, researchers at Harvard University in 1996 found that eating and talking together at mealtimes was more effective at developing children's vocabulary than play or story time.

Stimulating and engaging conversation, feeling listened to and valued are important for improved mood and prolonged mental acuity. Put simply, our minds stay younger if they are active and engaged – and what better way to engage than around the supper table.

USING SUPPLEMENTS

Double Nobel Prize winner Dr Linus Pauling said, "You can trace every disease, every sickness and every ailment to a mineral deficiency."

Your body uses macronutrients (fat, protein, carbohydrate and fibre) for growth, maintenance and repair. It uses micronutrients (vitamins and minerals, as well as enzymes and so on) to work at a cellular level to nourish you down to your smallest molecule.

In an ideal world we would get all the nutrients we need from the foods that we eat. But modern food practices (including the ways in which our foods are grown, farmed, transported and cooked) are far removed from the ideals that enable us to gain all the nourishment, nutrients, minerals and satisfaction we need from our food. For example, tomatoes and lettuces are picked young and shipped in cold storage in order to appear idyllic on the store shelves, without giving the plants enough time to ripen properly and so gain all the nutritional value that they could.

Of course, if you're following my principles of eating farm-fresh foods, in as natural a state as possible, you are already doing the best you can do to make sure the food on your plate is as nutrient-dense as it can be. Sadly, though, it's often still not enough. Even if we were to eat the recommended eight servings of fruit and vegetables a day, picked straight from the garden, most of us would still be nutritionally depleted in one or more areas – simply because our soils aren't as rich and nourishing as they used to be.

So, in order to plug the gap, we sometimes need to look to supplements. I suggest you keep a food diary for a week or two and check it against a list of essential vitamins and minerals, antioxidants and essential fats to see where you might best benefit from supplements and which nutrients you want them to contain. However, are all supplements as good as each other? No!

When you swallow a multi-vitamin, most specifically a tablet, the active ingredients are supposed to be released to your stomach and then pass through the small intestine where they are absorbed into your bloodstream. Most supplements, however, don't do the job. Acids in the stomach destroy nutrients from poor-quality tablets, which means that your body isn't really absorbing anything very much of any value. If you choose the wrong supplement, you most likely will end up with nothing other than expensive pee (sorry to be blunt about it!). Unfortunately, the supplement industry isn't regulated, which means that the quality of the supplements available varies widely. Producing a high-quality supplement does not simply involve mixing the various ingredients and packaging them together. Creating supplements involves a scientific formulation of nature's synergy into a single dose. When created by skilled scientists, such a supplement is far greater than the sum of its parts. Not only are these supplements combined properly, but they are also more bio-available, which means they are readily available to be used by the body.

Here are my top tips for getting your supplements right:

- Make sure the nutrients in your supplements are not
  isolated. There isn't a single food source in nature that
  contains a nutrient in isolation – individual nutrients are
  part of a complex food matrix designed to deliver that
  nutrient to your body in the most effective way possible.
  A vitamin C supplement, for example, is not effectively
  absorbed into your body unless it contains the other
  nutrients (ascorbinogen, bioflavonoids, rutin and so on)
  that are present in naturally vitamin-C-rich food. These
  are all vital parts of the delivery system that your body
  recognizes when trying to assimilate this vitamin. Similarly,
  in order for your body to absorb vitamin B12, it also needs
  a supply of folic acid (another B-vitamin). The relationship
  works the other way round, too – folic acid needs B12.
  If you take one of these nutrients without the other, your
  body doesn't reap the benefits. So, when you are choosing
  a supplement, find one that provides vitamins, minerals
  and fats that are combined as they are in nature – most
  manufacturers will shout about the fact if their products are
  naturally combined. If you're uncertain, ask for advice from
  a qualified nutritionist.
- Choose cold-pressed supplements. Heating nutrients to over
  115°C frazzles the enzymes so they no longer nourish your
  body. If it doesn't say "cold pressed" on the packaging, don't
  buy it.
- For powdered supplements (including those in capsules),
  choose the vegan option, even if you yourself aren't vegan.
  Other forms can contain nasty chemicals.
- Read the ingredients for signs of bulking agents or fillers,
  such as petrochemicals that were never intended for human
  consumption! If you see anything suspicious, think again.
  Choose supplements that are only nutrients, nothing more,
  nothing less. If in doubt, Google the words you don't
  understand before you buy.

- Don't assume that if you pay more, you're necessarily getting better quality. Make sure you read the packaging carefully and you understand what all the ingredients are and what they do.
- Beware of supplements that claim they provide way more than the recommended daily allowance (RDA) for that nutrient. You don't need the extra, so why choose a supplement that over-delivers? It's just a ploy to get you to spend extra money on manufactured alternatives that you don't need.

Easy supplements

Supplements don't only come in tablet form, however. You can buy them in powder or oil form from reputable sources and add them to meals or your daily smoothie to give yourself a fantastic boost. Here are a few superfood supplements that I take myself daily and highly recommend:

Cold-pressed hemp
Wheatgrass
Barley grass
Spirulina
Maca
Raw cacao

These can be easily put into cereals, juices or smoothies. We need these nutrients at all stages of our lives because all of the cells of your body need oxygen, water and nutrients. These superfoods can contain up to 400 percent better nutritional value than most foods that people are consuming today.

I believe nature holds all the answers and that boosting your diet with additional nutrients will further boost your health and vitality. Make sure any supplements you take are organic and raw so that they contain the live enzymes. Remember, nutrition doesn't need to be complicated and our nutritional needs don't necessarily change because we age. Just listen to your body and use common sense – as long as you are getting good amounts of the essential vitamins and minerals, you'll be nourishing your cells well and optimizing your potential for living forever young.

> **We're an upright column of walking ocean water. Walk barefoot, touch the earth and eat foods that are rich in antioxidants, calcium and magnesium.**
>
> David "Avocado" Wolfe – author,
> superfood and nutrition expert

WATER: THE SOURCE OF ALL LIFE

No chapter on the secrets of how to nourish your body would be complete without looking at water. All living things – from seaweed to humans – need water for survival. I'll be straight with you, folks: if life can't exist without water, then your longevity can't be possible without water, either.

Do you remember the first secret, "Breathe" – to oxygenate your body properly? If you do, you know that you could live only approximately three minutes without oxygen and only three days without water – this is much less time than you can survive without food.

About 70 percent of the planet is covered in water and between 55 and 70 percent of your body is made of water (the actual amount depends upon gender, age and weight). That's how important water is to survival. You need it for healthy blood, lymph, detoxification, digestion, skin, eyes and hair. Dizziness, muscle spasm, cramp, bone pain, dry eyes, dry skin, reduced immunity, headaches, memory loss and dry mouth are all signs that your body is crying out for water – along with reduced urine output and yellow urine, of course. If you lose a mere 10 percent of water from your body, you can suffer severe dehydration; and according to some sources, if you lose up to 20 percent you are at risk of death. That's pretty mind-blowing.

How much water do you need?

You need to aim for between eight and ten glasses of water every day to keep your body functioning optimally, plus an extra three or four glasses if you've been working out, to replace the fluids you will have lost through sweat.

It is worth noting, though, that water is water – not other liquids that contain water, such as fizzy or caffeinated drinks, and not alcohol, which all have well-documented negative effects on the body. For example:

- Caffeine is a xanthine alkaloid – a psychoactive stimulant drug that affects the central nervous system to temporarily alleviate drowsiness and restore wakefulness.
- Coffee is an acidic food – and we already know that the body should be slightly alkaline. One cup of coffee or a couple of cups of tea are not harmful, but heavy caffeine use can cause headache, jitteriness, lack of concentration and dehydration.
- Alcohol (even in moderation) negatively affects every system in your body, which, of course, is not good for longevity. Furthermore, by stripping your skin and hair of water and nutrients, impeding your ability to sleep well, and leading to weight gain, the ageing effects of drinking alcohol are not just going on inside your body. If you want to live forever young, the best advice I can give is complete abstention – but I accept that's not necessarily realistic. Try cutting down gradually, with the aim of limiting your intake to only two or three units a week.

"No alcohol, no coffee, no fizzy drinks! But plain water is just so boring!" I hear you say. So, try to jazz it up a bit. You could try replacing sugar-laden cordials with water laced with a squeeze of lemon, or flavoured with some cucumber and mint. Herbal teas and diluted fruit juice are another good alternative. Milk can count towards your daily limit, but every glass of milk counts only as half a glass of water.

Finally, increase your intake of water-rich foods in your diet with fresh fruits and vegetables. The waters in these will help to hydrate you, which is like giving yourself a cleansing, refreshing, nourishing shower from within.

Water for your spirit

Chew on this: the only reason why life on Earth is possible is because of water. Thus far, it seems that our watery planet is unique in the solar system. However, as well as being a physical necessity, water has the power to enhance us spiritually, too. In fact, water has been a metaphor for the spirit in cultures across the world since time immemorial.

Bruce Lee once said "be like water" because water can take on so many different forms. Sometimes it's solid like ice, sometimes it evaporates into thin air; sometimes it flows through and around rocks in streams; sometimes it rains down from the sky to nourish the earth; and sometimes it flows in great oceans and creates waves full of power and energy.

Think about how those differing properties of water could become metaphors in your own life:

- Be solid in your relationships and your belief in yourself and those around you.
- Be light and ethereal by casting off concerns and living in the present.
- Be flowing and creative when you encounter obstacles in your path.

- Be nourishing in your interactions with others, and take time to nourish yourself.
- Gather your power and energy and "make waves" of positive change in your life.

The late Japanese author, researcher and photographer Masaru Emoto (1943–2014) believed that our thoughts and emotions affect the water in our body and mind. And he set out to prove it. He projected certain intentions into different receptacles of water, then froze each one and took pictures of the ice crystals. If the thoughts were pure and positive, such as love, peace, thank you and so on, the frozen water crystals were symmetrical and looked like beautiful snowflakes. Every time the intentions were negative, such as I hate you, you make me sick, shut up and so on, the crystals were imbalanced and irregular. Although his research is the subject of much criticism, the notion that the way we think and feel can affect the "flow" (of energy, of positivity, of attitude) through our body and mind is not unusual – it is an underlying principle of ancient philosophies from India to Meso-America. If we think of this life-energy as the water that we need so fundamentally to live, then even if we don't believe in the science of Emoto's findings, we can certainly live by his ethos.

Try it now: The power of water*

So, if water is a metaphor for spirit and flow, it makes the perfect subject for a meditation or visualization. Try the two exercises below. The first is a visualization and the second a three-minute meditation. Practise them as » often as you can – connecting yourself to the purity and power of water. It can be particularly useful to do this exercise in the morning – to help you start off your day positively and with a strong intention for good "flow".

Improving your inner flow

- Pour yourself a glass of water. Before you drink it, look at it and project into it positive thoughts and energy. Think of this like the blessing you made for your food – only this time you're doing it for the water you're about to drink. Be thankful for it, consider its life-giving properties (for your body, for the plants in your garden, for all the animals on the Earth) and marvel at how this simple, clear liquid can hold such power.

- Now take your first sip. Be really mindful about the feeling of the water on your lips and tongue, and as it flows down your throat. Imagine it flowing into all parts of your body – through your veins, into your heart and mind. Remind yourself how it is imbued with positive energy and really feel that energy flowing through you.

- Keeping sipping and imagine the water cleansing your whole system. As it flushes out the impurities in your body, feel a sense of calm wash through you. Be thankful for the sense of peace and tranquility this brings. Really focus on the flow – imagine it in your toes, your calves, your thighs, through your abdomen, your heart and chest, down your arms into your fingers and all the way to the top of your head. Calm washes through you.

»

The mind as a pool of water

Another analogy that really helps me is to imagine my mind like a pool of water. When that pool is muddled and stressed, the pool is murky and muddy. However, when my mind is still and calm, the water is still and calm and in it I can see perfectly reflected thoughts, memories and imaginings. If you learn to still the waters of your mind, clarity will follow.

Here's a simple three-minute meditation to help calm the "pool of water" in your mind. Enjoy taking this time out and feel the difference in just three minutes:

- Take in a deep breath as you relax into your body, hold it, and exhale.
- Take in another deep breath and feel yourself relaxing, unwinding and letting go of anything that doesn't serve you.
- Now continue to breathe deeply and rhythmically and imagine yourself being the drop in the ocean that becomes the ocean, expanding your awareness.
- Understand there is more to your wonder than you've experienced so far. By believing that you are more powerful than you think, you can relax knowing that you are exactly where you are meant to be right now.
- You are doing great at what you're doing so give yourself a break.
- Trust that life has got your back and can see a bigger vision for you – a vision where you get to be all you came here to be. One where you can flow like water, shine like the sun, weather the different seasons and be in alignment with greater forces that surround you. »

> • Recognize that by following the secrets in this book you are aiming to be the best version of you that allows love, positive energy, peace and creativity to flood out of your being and into all aspects of your life.

NOW YOU CAN BE NOURISHED

Changes to your nutritional choices don't need to be drastic – and, in fact, in order to make them sustainable, baby steps are a much better way to go. Over time, you can transform your diet into something that truly nourishes you from within. I hope throughout this chapter you've learned how minimizing toxins, improving healthy nutrients, and feeding your body life-giving water not only gives your physical self what it needs for longevity, but (especially when we look at the symbolic meanings of water) improve the functioning of your mind and spirit, too.

LIVING FOREVER YOUNG
TOP 10 TAKEAWAYS: NOURISH

- Aim to eat meat only two or three times each week, or fewer if you can, even give it up altogether.
- Reduce your dairy intake, or even give it up altogether.
- Eat a rainbow of fruits and vegetables to ensure you're getting a whole range of antioxidant nutrients, which keep your body's cells healthy.
- Choose organic meat, fruit and vegetables – using as much organic produce as you can afford.
- Avoid weight-loss diets and instead opt for healthy choices

and natural balance – you will meet your natural weight that way and won't need to go for a fad.

- Give thanks for the nourishment available to you – quietly or formally be grateful for the food you eat and those who share it with you.
- Use supplements and superfoods exactly as they were intended – to supplement your healthy diet – and always make sure they are the best quality, natural supplements and superfoods you can afford, in natural combinations.
- Drink water every day in its freshest and purest form – your body's cells need water more than they need food!
- Clear your mind using water as a metaphor for something clear and still – like a still pool of water.
- Learn to flow like water in your life – around obstacles and through tributaries in your life, always aiming for your goal or purpose.

OVER TO YOU

Now that you've read the bulk of this chapter, it's time for you to choose how exactly you are going to make the secrets of good nourishing *your own* by integrating them into your daily life. So...

- Close the book and consider the ways in which you would feel most able and happy to start putting this chapter's suggestions, or any other nourishing-related ideas of your own that you have, into practice.
- Then take a pen and notebook or piece of paper and write down the three, or five, of these ways that you most like the idea of really committing to, and that you feel will not only be really useful for you, but also achievable and sustainable. For example, you might decide to have a fresh green juice

every morning to kick off your day; start keeping a bottle or jug of water on your desk and setting an alarm to drink a glass every hour; go on a nice weekly trip to your local farmer's market instead of buying all your fruit and veg from the local supermarket; or research and invest in quality supplements to ensure your body is getting all the nutrients it needs.

- If the thought of three or five things overwhelms you, just start with one – baby steps are the best way to go and as long as you keep up what you have started you'll soon find momentum building and you will want to, and be able to, do more.

- If you need a little help and encouragement to get into this decision-making zone, try the "Lost in Music" technique on page xxi to set you on your way.

- Then read your chosen action points out loud to yourself – and make an inward commitment about how, when and where you're going to start putting them into practice – as of this week, or even *today* if possible. Feel free to write these practical details beneath the action points if you feel it will help you stick at them...

- Now use this list as your personal guide to enhancing the "Nourish" section of your life-balance wheel, coming back to the list any time you feel the need to revise it or add to it...

WHERE ARE YOU NOW? (PART 2)

Once you have been using the above list of action points for about a month, it will be time to assess how things are going. So – remember that list of statements you rated at the start of the chapter? Well, read and rate them again (I've listed them below, so that you don't have to flick back).

Please score the following questions for nourishing on a scale of 1 to 10, with 1 being "not at all true for me" and 10 being "completely true for me".

- I am aware of my diet and try to eat healthily every day.
- I look forward to preparing and make all my main meals from scratch.
- I eat foods that sustain my energy levels all day, rather than relying on caffeine or sugar.
- I take combined, natural supplements and superfoods only as a safeguard to fill any gaps in my healthy diet.
- I make sure that I drink at least two litres of quality alkaline water a day, more when I exercise.

Your ultimate aim in terms of a score is 40 or above – an 80 percent plus result that shows you have this secret nailed and are really using it to help you live forever young. Keep pushing yourself, however, and do what you can to avoid being complacent and slipping back into bad habits.

If you're implementing the takeaways and practising your chosen action points/techniques, I hope you'll see that your score has improved since the first time you did it.

If you're not quite where you want to be, return to the "Over to you" section in order to revisit your key action points and ensure that they still feel relevant to you (see page xx for more advice on revisiting and reassessing your goals).

After you have been practising your new "Nourish" techniques for a while, don't forget to revisit your life-balance wheel at some stage (see page xxii) to keep track of progress in terms of how you feel in this area of your life. This will help you to acknowledge your achievements and to keep making further progress. The more you shade in every segment, the bigger the steps you are making along your path of living forever young!

SECRET 4: REST

Let me ask you a question: do you drive? And if you do drive, do you have your own car? Assuming yes, do you look after it – fill it up with petrol, top up the radiator with water regularly, give it an oil change every so often, pop it into the garage for a full service? Of course, you do – because your car has to be roadworthy.

Now, think about your own vehicle, your body. When was the last time you gave it some love and attention? What about your mind? No car can keep going well without it being serviced – it might keep running, but not as smoothly as it would if you showed it a bit of love every now and then. The same applies to your body and your mind.

The great thing is you don't get any servicing bills with your body. Rest, recuperation and a little bit of homemade pampering are all that it needs to feel rejuvenated – as long as you do so regularly. Like all marvellous machines, your body needs to be able to rest in order to function optimally long into your old age – you wouldn't drive a car continually and expect it to last over 100 years. Don't expect the same of your body and mind.

The natural way we rest is through sleep, but is sleep all we need to live forever young? And what ageing effects do lack of rest and lack of sleep have on your body? In this chapter we'll look at the importance of rest and sleep and how to make sure we get enough of both to protect your body and mind long into old age.

But, before you begin, let's look at where you are with your rest right now.

WHERE ARE YOU NOW? (PART 1)

Please score the following questions for resting on a scale of 1 to 10, with 1 being "not at all true for me" and 10 being "completely true for me". Note down your score. Then, when you've completed this chapter and implemented its advice, try the questions again.

- I wake up every day feeling rested and ready for the day ahead of me.
- I rarely have energy dips. My energy levels remain constant all day.
- I fall asleep easily when I go to bed and wake up energized.
- I take regular "time out" from my daily life to really rest and recuperate, such as an hour a week, or two or three weekends a year.
- I use meditation, visualization or other relaxation methods every day as a means to rest and still my mind.

THE NEED FOR REST AND SLEEP

The body cannot function without rest, and specifically without sleep. We know this because it's impossible to fight sleep interminably – eventually, the body takes over and sleep ensues. So, although there is still much that baffles scientists about the nature of rest and sleep, one thing is certain – we can't do without them.

Interestingly, scientists have shown that rest – that is, complete, uninterrupted, unstimulated switching off with your eyes closed – is almost as restorative as sleep. If you started walking one day, even at the slowest pace possible, with the intention of just keeping going, eventually your muscles would tire to the point that they give way. You would have to stop. Rest, then, is a time of repair and renewal, just as sleep is. It does most of the jobs that sleep does, but at a slightly lower level, while we are awake. Sleep, on the other hand, is the brain's prescription for complete mental and physical recovery. Scientists think that sleep is a time not only for the physical body to repair and rejuvenate, but for the mind to consolidate the day, process learning and form memories. However, sleep scientists also believe that meditation – resting with your eyes closed, but remaining awake – is pretty good for mental decluttering, too.

As we age, our needs for rest change – think how a baby sleeps for most of the day and night. By our early 20s, our need for sleep dramatically drops, with most young adults needing only between eight and ten hours a night. In middle age our sleep needs are relatively stable – with most adults needing between six and eight hours a night. Then, in our twilight years, changes in the body clock and hormone levels mean that both men and women sleep less – often getting between four and six hours a night; although in old age, we tend to fall asleep early and wake up very early. During sleep (or rest) the body has time to repair and regenerate. All your systems work together to keep you healthy without the distraction of being awake. When you think about it, it makes perfect sense.

Studies show that getting the right amount of restorative sleep and rest every day is fundamental to stemming some of the key signs of ageing. For example, lack of sleep has been linked with:

- poor skin and hair health;
- reduced memory function;
- increased risk of heart disease;
- increased risk of some cancers, including age-related cancers such as breast cancer and prostate cancer;

- increased risk of low mood and depression;
- tendency towards weight gain and obesity;
- increased risk of joint pain;
- increased risk of Type-II diabetes.

Importantly, then, we need to give our body that self-care that comes from improving sleep quality and getting appropriate amounts of rest. When we sleep the body rests and recovers – it's that simple. When we don't get enough rest we risk burnout, break down (physically, mentally and emotionally) and age faster. So how do we improve our sleep and rest?

THE PROCESS OF SLEEP

Before we look at how to improve the quality of your sleep, I want to take a bit of time to explain the nature and process of sleep and rest in physiological terms, so that you can see just how everything is interconnected.

The main regulator for sleep is your circadian rhythm – that's the 24-hour in-built biological clock that tells your body what time of day or night it is. All your cells live by this rhythm, from the cells in your reproductive system to the cells in your brain. The key to the rhythm when it comes to your sleep is the presence (or not) of light, which triggers hormone fluctuations in your body that make you feel sleepy or bring you to wakefulness.

The most important hormone for your sleep rhythm is melatonin. Secreted by the pineal gland in your brain, melatonin does not cause sleep in itself, but is a messenger for your brain to indicate when darkness is falling, triggering the cascade of sleepiness. Levels of melatonin rise steadily through the night, peaking at about 3 or 4am, when they start to tail off again as dawn breaks.

Once we are asleep, sleep itself is characterized by the "sleep cycle". In healthy adults, this is a roughly 90-minute cycle that takes us through two major types of sleep (dreaming and non-dreaming), known as R and N sleep respectively, with N sleep subdivided into three further periods or "stages" – N1, N2 and N3 – which are drowsy, light and deep sleep. The whole cycle of R and N sleep is repeated four or five times a night to make up your eight-ish hours.

Interestingly, and significantly for your health and well-being, not every cycle contains stages of the same length. So, at the start of the night, when you are most tired you'll spend most time in N3 (really deep sleep – the kind that makes you really hard to wake up) and the least time in N2 (light sleep) and R (dreaming) sleep. The last 90-minute cycle is usually made up of the least N3 sleep and the most N1 and R sleep of the night.

It's during N3 sleep that your body does the most work, rebuilding and repairing muscles, fighting infection and consolidating all the mental effort you've made during the day. Your body is so clever that if you have periods of too little sleep, when you do get the chance for some slumber, rather than you sleeping longer overall, you'll simply spend more time over the course of the night in N3 than you might have done if you'd had consistently good sleep in the preceding days. In other words, it's a myth to think that you need to get more hours' kip if you've been a bit sleep deprived – it's the quality of the sleep, not the quantity, that will set you straight.

THE PURPOSE OF SLEEP

Scientists are still pretty hazy on the precise purpose of sleep. But we do know that there are certain physiological processes that work more efficiently when we're asleep than when we're awake. Not only that, common sense tells us that because we have to sleep (remember, it's impossible to stay awake indefinitely), whatever sleep is for, it matters!

Here are some of the benefits that getting enough good sleep brings us:

- Sleep encourages **cell repair, growth and healing** – during sleep, studies show that the body is better at strengthening bone and repairing muscle damage. Not only that – it also helps repair and replenish skin cells. If you want to live forever young, you need healthy bones, healthy organs and healthy muscles that give you good movement and flexibility, and youthful-looking skin. Studies show that the uppermost layers of our skin are better able to repair themselves from skin damage and dehydration if we are getting good amounts of restful sleep every night. And don't forget that the appearance of dark circles and bags under your eyes is the result of the blood vessels in the fine skin dilating, and releasing liquid that gives you that ageing, puffy look.

- Sleep enables your **brain cells to replenish their energy stores**, helping to make sure that we have enough energy up there to keep those brain cells firing all day. It also ensures that we consolidate our memories fully and helps to relieve stress and therefore improve mental function. So when you've rested properly, this helps keeps your brain younger. The flip side of this is when you wake up after a poor night's sleep with a foggy head, inability to focus properly and tasks take longer to complete.

- Sleep increases levels of the **human growth hormone** (HGH) – this is probably one of the reasons why babies sleep so much (after all, they have lots of growing to do!). For adults, it means that the body has the opportunity to repair and replenish cells in the vital organs, as well as the muscles, skin and hair.

- Sleep **protects your heart** – research shows that those who lack sufficient amounts of sleep have higher levels of stress hormone circulating in their body, which puts additional strain on your heart. Even worse than that, some studies show that through affecting the body's immune system, lack of sleep or poor sleep quality can speed up the hardening of the arteries associated with old age – which means the heart has to pump harder to get the blood around the body. Keeping your heart beating strong and full of love are key ingredients for you to maintain health and vitality – in other words, to live forever young.

- Sleep **enables your immune system** to do its work fighting infection. Manufacture of both T-helper cells and cytotoxic T cells, which are essential disease-fighting soldiers in your body, appears to increase during sleep. If you don't get enough sleep, bacteria and viruses have more chance of taking hold. Furthermore, preliminary research suggests that those who work shifts (and so suffer disrupted sleep patterns and are often in sleep debt) are up to 30 percent more likely to develop certain cancers, including breast cancer for women and prostate cancer for men. The theory is that the interruption to the biological clock encourages cell mutation at a faster rate than those who don't work shifts – and cell mutation can lead to more rapid tumour growth. However, if you are one of these people who only get a few hours sleep, don't worry – one way in which you can boost your sleep benefit is by clearly setting your intention before you fall asleep. Imagine yourself waking refreshed, rebuilt and recovered enough for your needs the next day. See yourself with enough energy and vigour to handle the challenges of the day. By programming your mind this way, you take back control to be able to achieve this!

- Sleep **improves muscle memory** – that is, your body's ability to remember the sequence of movements you need to make in order to achieve a particular physical activity. If you think in terms of being forever young, this means that during sleep your body consolidates the memories of the muscle movements that give you your suppleness. Want to be athletic into old age? Get some good sleep!

On the flip side…

- Lack of sleep dramatically **impedes your coordination**, judgement and reaction times. You've probably already heard that driving while sleep-deprived is like driving when drunk – one study suggests that getting in a car to drive after being awake for 18 hours without resting is like driving with a blood alcohol limit of 0.05, where 0.08 is considered "drunk".
- Lack of sleep makes us feel more ratty and emotional. Ever felt miserable after a bout of poor sleep? Ever felt **tired and emotional** and said "It's just because I'm tired." Of course! This is because you haven't reset yourself with proper sleep – it's like recharging your phone and having a power cut in the night so you only got charged 50%. Then you can only use your phone effectively for half the amount of time, and this is the same with your mind and your body. (A quick remedy for this is taking a few minutes out during the day to practise a short mindfulness exercise – these tend to have a fantastically restorative effect of bringing you back up to speed when tiredness hits, see page 95).
- Lack of sleep **impairs the body's ability to respond to insulin levels** in the blood. Insulin is the hormone that tells your body when to release sugar into your bloodstream for energy. If that communication mechanism breaks down, the body stores sugar as fat, rather than using it up – and you'll feel more tired, which often leads to sugary quick-fix eating. In addition, sleep helps us maintain a healthy weight. This

is because it moderates and balances the levels of hormones leptin and ghrelin, which are responsible for suppressing appetite when we're full and stimulating appetite when we're hungry, respectively.

• Lack of sleep affects your testosterone levels. If you are a man and want a **sex drive** worthy of your younger self it's probably worth knowing that a study published in 2011 found that sleep deprivation can age your testosterone production by 15 years. In fact, testosterone levels are affected in women, too – so, when the mood is more "No, darling, not tonight, I'm tired", go with it – because nothing will get better in the bedroom department if you don't get enough sleep in the first place!

PUTTING YOUR SLEEP RIGHT

There are so many reasons why we might not get all the sleep we need for our body to function optimally – stress, work patterns, overstimulation, eating too late and lots of other reasons can mean that, even when we go to bed at a good time, the sleep that follows isn't restful or restorative and has the opposite effect to living forever young. So, what can you do? Here are my top tips:

• Stop doing mentally demanding work at least 60 minutes before you go to bed – give your brain time to calm down before you try to sleep. Ideally, stop all stimulation, if you can – including the TV.

• Try to have your heaviest meal at lunchtime, rather than in the evening, if you can. At the very least, try to eat more than four hours before bedtime. That way, your body goes to sleep with your food already digested, so that your energy can be directed to sleep and repair, rather than to breaking down your last meal.

- Avoid caffeine and alcohol before bedtime. Aim to have your last caffeinated drink at midday (it can take up to six hours for your body to work the caffeine through your system). And there's no such thing as a worthwhile alcoholic nightcap. Alcohol stimulates your system, so while it might seem that it makes you sleepy at the start of the night, you're more likely to wake during the night or to sleep fitfully if you drink late in the evening and/or before bed.

- Limit evening screen time – and by that I mean not just the TV (as I've already mentioned), but also computer, smartphone and tablet time. Most hand-held devices are backlit, which means that bright, often blue, light is pinging its way into your optic nerves, preventing the production of melatonin (the hormone that tells your body it's time for sleeping).

- Create a bedtime routine to get your mind in the mood for sleep. You might start by writing down a list of things you've achieved in the day, and a list of things you need to achieve tomorrow (celebrating your successes and organizing your next steps). Then, perhaps try a 10-minute peaceful meditation or visualization (such as the one on page 95), followed by a cleansing ritual (perhaps washing your hands and face, and brushing your teeth), before you get into bed. If you do the same things in the same order every night, you prepare your body and mind to go to sleep. Note that if you want to have a nighttime bath or shower, make sure it's at least 90 minutes before you intend to go to bed – your body needs to cool down to fall asleep. A bath or shower is a good idea, but only if you give yourself time to lose the heat so, cool or cold showers can be great if you feel up to it.

- Try to get to bed at roughly the same time every night, and get up at roughly the same time every morning, even at the weekends or when you have days off. Your body clock likes predictability. Even if you have an exceptional late night, for a party, say, try to get up at the usual time the following morning. Your body will make back the sleep deficit in increased deep sleep, rather than in hours.

- Remember that your body clock is set by the changes in light – so dim the lights before bedtime and take steps to keep your bedroom nice and dark. Use blackout blinds or heavy curtains to block out street lighting.

- Keep your bedroom cool – we sleep better when we're cooler rather than when we're warmer (and in fact rapidly falling internal body temperature is one of the ways in which your brain knows its time for sleep). Use layers on your bed, with sheets and blankets, so that you can lose or add layers if you are too warm or cool during the night. In the same vein, try to use cotton bedding and cotton nightclothes – cotton wicks away sweat, to keep your body at the perfect temperature for sleep.

THE POWER OF YOUR DREAMS

One of the unique features of sleep is dreaming. We don't dream when we're awake, so what are dreams for? Some people believe that dreams are the mind's way of processing the events of the day, in weird and wonderful manifestations of our real lives. Others believe they are for consolidating or managing events from our past. The truth is that we don't know for certain – all we really know about dreams is that we all have them. When you wake up thinking you haven't had a dream that's probably not true – it's just that you woke up a while since your last period of dreaming sleep. When you wake up remembering your dream, you have probably just had it, or were in it when you woke.

Keeping a dream diary is one way that you could start to see if there is a pattern to your dreams and try to assess what (if anything) they are trying to teach you. Keep a notebook

beside your bed and when you wake write down everything
you can remember about your dreams from the night before –
in as much detail as possible. After a month of recording your
dreams in this way, have a look back and consider whether you
can spot any patterns in them – recurring events or people, or
moods or feelings. Could they be a window to your spirit?

THE VALUE OF REST

So, all that's sleep – but is that the same as rest? And if not,
how can we get some of that too? I like to think of rest as the
complete letting go of mental chatter and outside distraction
in order to still and calm down the mind. It's important
for staying forever young, because it not only gives your
body some time to regenerate and regroup, but it also gives
your mind time to consolidate and refocus. Good-quality
downtime has been proven time and again to improve mood
and cognitive function, and relieve stress and anxiety. Imagine
what it's like to be lying on a beach completely immersed in
the sounds of the waves against the shore – nothing else, just
that sound filling your mind. Or, if the beach isn't your thing,
imagine lying on warm grass and filling your mind with the
sound of the breeze through the trees, or birdsong. To me,
being able to fill my mind with only what is happening in the
here and now is true rest.

I suppose what I'm really talking about is mindfulness
– paying attention to the present moment with a good
intention and without being distracted by anything other
than your experience of the present. You don't even have to be
completely still to practise mindfulness – walking meditations,
t'ai chi and yoga are all moving practices that encourage you
to focus completely on the act and sensations of what you
are doing in any particular moment without distraction. And

if your mind wanders during any mindful practice, as it is bound to, don't worry – simply bring it back to the focus of your attention and carry on.

Meditation plays a big role in slowing down the aging process. In that deep state of restfulness the body can throw off accumulated stress.

Thom Knoles –
Maharishi of Vedic meditation

Try it now: Mindfulness meditation*

If you've never practised mindfulness before, it can be helpful to start with a visualization to get yourself used to the notion of emptying your mind of its chatter and focusing on something specific. It can also help to make a visualization a regular part of your sleep routine, to help tune your mind and body into the notion of going to sleep. Or, you can use it simply to find an inner space that takes you away from reality and stress and into a place of deep, but waking calm. The following is one of my favourite visualizations – try it for yourself.

- Find somewhere quiet and sit or lie comfortably. Position yourself so that you have no reason to get distracted by any aches or pains.
- Close your eyes and focus on your breathing. Feel the breath coming in through your nose, and out through your mouth. Spend a few moments settling into a steady rhythm.

»

- Now, beginning at your feet, cast your mind from toe to top – notice any areas of tension in your body. When you do, don't just move on, but stop and breathe into that area. With your out-breath, imagine that you let the tension go. Don't apply any force to the out-breath, just a gentle release. Keep going until you've released the tense spots throughout your body.

- When you're feeling fully relaxed, take a mental journey. Imagine yourself barefoot, opening a gate into a peaceful garden. Notice the scent of fresh grass and flowers, listen to the birds chirping, feel the softness of the warm, summer breeze across your face. What else can you smell, hear and feel? Really try to capture the image of the garden in all its glory. What's the weather like? What can you feel underfoot? Can you identify different birdsongs?

- When you're ready, close the gate behind you and imagine stepping onto a path. Visualize yourself taking one step at a time towards the sound of rushing water – with every step the sound gets louder. Soon, you can see a beautiful waterfall up ahead. The water cascades downwards into a clear, deep pool.

- Imagine walking to the edge of the pool. You dip the toe of one foot into the water – how does it feel? Try to think beyond just the temperature – is it soft or harsh? Silky or icy? Can you see the bottom of the pool, or is it so deep as to appear totally black?

- Beside the pool is a mound of mossy grass – laid out like a soft, earth bed. You lie down on the mound.

»

- How does it feel? Imagine its soft, sponginess supporting and enveloping you. The sound of the water nearby is soothing, the air is cool and fresh. You feel totally relaxed. Stay in this place for a few minutes and then gently bring yourself back to your present reality, refreshed and re-energized and ready to re-engage with your day.

This visualization is something that helps me totally empty my mind and immerse myself in tranquillity. Of course, for you the sound of water might be a distraction or you might find it too energizing. If so, that's fine – think of your own most relaxing place and make that the subject of your visualization. As long as you are able to immerse yourself in the image in your mind, without being distracted by outside thoughts or stressful feelings, you can properly disconnect from real life and give your body and mind space and time to recharge.

A change is as good as a rest

A 2015 study released by the American Psychological Association concluded that holidays are a great way to manage stress because they separate us from our normal routine – the routine that, in whatever ways, causes stress in the first place. So, while we might talk of rest as a daily moment of escape, time for meditation, visualization or simple tranquillity, it is also the ability to leave behind daily life and discover new places, new experiences and even new people, and to be the best, most natural version of your self without the trappings of normal life. Of course, you don't necessarily need a long holiday – an afternoon spent in a museum, exploring a nature trail, building sandcastles on a local beach, a concert of your favourite music… all these take us away from the humdrum of our everyday lives. Think about how children react when you tell them they're going to go on holiday – they're excited and energized, as I hope we would be as adults, too. Holidays plug into our childlike innocent view of the world where we get to go on an adventure. They keep us young and playful and full of wonder.

Letting go of long-held anxiety

We all collect sadness or disappointment in our lives – it's inevitable. Even if we have developed a positive mindset, which enables us to see the light beyond a deep sadness, we often carry internal scars and, whether we realize it or not, these do affect our present day. On my retreats, I use deep relaxation techniques to encourage my clients to let go of long-held anxiety or pain and to reinvent themselves, looking and feeling younger and with a greater zest for life. It's amazing – you can see the years fall away as all those lines of sadness are let go. Relaxation is powerful, but *letting go* of whatever isn't serving you is the key.

A simple illustration: imagine what a child is like when they want an ice-cream and you initially say no – they usually turn into either an expert negotiator or a huge pain. That ice-cream is really important to them and they cling on to the idea of it. If you then say they can have it, all their problems seem to disappear in an instant – they let go of that problem, their world changes, and they feel better. This is what I want for you. It is essential to let go of whatever you're holding onto that isn't serving you for you to progress on your journey of living forever young.

It's a true story...

Deep relaxation is one of the key elements of my retreats.
And it can have dramatic effects. A lady arrived at the retreat
holding on to a broken heart that she'd had for about 40
years. A relationship breakdown that had occurred in her
distant past had affected her so much that she had built
up a protection mechanism around her heart – allowing it
to remain broken and keeping it hidden from experiencing
real love again. Step by step, I guided her through a deep
relaxation process that enabled her to bring her broken heart
to the surface and to let it go. With that immense release,
her face immediately changed – when she came out of the
relaxation, she literally looked ten years younger and she
had new vigour and energy. When she arrived on the retreat
she had been expecting to go home and end her present
relationship – but her new lease of life, and her release as
a result of deep relaxation, enabled her to find confidence,
belief and connection with her partner, and they now live
happily together today.

Find your best rest

If being exhausted and at the end of your tether makes you
think of an inviting warm bath full of rose petals or a candlelit,
pillow-filled room with soft music playing in the background,
then that's what you should go for, whenever you can. A short
spell of meditation works for me. Whatever your idea of a
good rest is, try to organize your life so you can fit in a bit of
downtime at least once a day. Try to rest your mind as well
as your body. You will definitely feel the benefit, and so will
those around you. I can't emphasize enough how just a short
period of switching off from the everyday will energize you and
relieve your stress, both of which are such key factors in living
forever young.

FINDING TIME FOR REST

Okay, I hear you. You're telling me that you're busy, that you don't have time for dedicated "resting" on top of working, exercising, cooking, cleaning, caring for your family, seeing your friends, connecting with your work colleagues and sleeping. I get it.

But what if I told you that just 15 minutes every day set aside for rest – time for you – would add up to a full 105 minutes of extra time that you have given your body and mind for recharging over the course of the week. You can do the maths yourself for the month and year – but I can assure you, it's significant. And really, 15 minutes isn't very much. I bet you spend at least 15 minutes a day on social media, or watching something fairly rubbish on television. I bet if you really trimmed at your life to make it as efficient as possible, you'd find significantly more than 15 minutes a day for rest and relaxation. Still, let's not jump the gun. Start small – find 5 minutes a day in the first week, then 10 minutes the next, then 15 minutes in the third. Once you've carved out your 15 minutes, keep it there. And keep it regular. With just a couple of weeks of practise it will become routine. Protect it – this is valuable, essential even, time for living forever young and you need it as much as you need the air that you breathe and the food that you eat.

Here are some ideas for how to carve out that 15 minutes extra a day:

- Over a week, become aware of how long you spend doing your everyday tasks and activities – perhaps jotting this down in a notebook. You'll soon be able to identify spaces in your day where you might block out 15 minutes to spend on yourself.
- Get up 15 minutes earlier – ideally, before anyone else in the house is up, so that this time feels special, exclusive and entirely yours.

- Ignore one chore each day – the washing load can wait, as can mopping the floor, or dusting the windowsills. Cleansing yourself is more important than cleansing your home. Postponing just one chore each day won't mean that the chores don't get done – you will probably find that you are more productive over the week having recharged yourself with a dedicated "rest" time anyway.
- Turn off your phone or the TV at a set time in the evening and take that opportunity to practise a short visualization or maybe a relaxing yoga stretch or move. You could even double-up with the yoga poses described in the Move chapter (see page 35) for this purpose.

NOW YOU CAN REST

So, if at the start of this chapter you were wondering why rest is a secret – after all, we all sleep – now you know that, in fact, it's not sleeping and resting themselves that are unknown to us, but the powerful effects they can have on your health and well-being, both physically, mentally and emotionally. Furthermore, you will have learned how to access more of your inner power through more effective rest and sleep that allows you to be fully recharged. All too often our modern world drives us into activity – to be better, faster, more brilliant, more accomplished. But, what if being better was just to be still. For me, restful stillness is the secret that makes everything else achievable. Calming your mind with good rest and sleep helps you see more clearly, think more clearly, let go of the stress and feel the good feelings – energy, positivity, vigour – that people living forever young experience everyday.

LIVING FOREVER YOUNG
TOP 10 TAKEAWAYS: REST

- Find 15 minutes every day for focused rest and relaxation – start small if you need to, just 5 minutes a day, building up until you've carved a full 15 minutes out of your day. Once you've found it, protect it.
- Create a bedtime routine, following the same pattern of activity in the hour before you go to bed every night.
- Try to go to bed at the same time every day and get up at the same time every morning, even on non-work days.
- Trust that your body will make back any sleep deficit if you give it the opportunity – you'll spend more time in deep sleep than in lighter phases of sleep, so don't panic if you have an exceptional late night.
- Before you go to bed, write down in a notebook the day's troubles and make a list of the things you have to do the following day. Put the notebook beside your bed safe in the knowledge that they will be there in the morning when you wake and they don't need to trouble you as you sleep.
- Make sure you get a regular change of scene – if it's not a holiday, take an afternoon to escape to a landscape that is unusual for you; or spend it in a museum or gallery.
- Your mind is better rested if it's fully in the present – not worrying about the past or future. Try to live each day mindfully, engaging in the present moment and giving it your full attention.
- Eat and drink in a way that supports your sleep – avoid alcohol and caffeine late at night, and try to eat your supper more than four hours before you go to bed.
- Keep your bedroom cool and dark so that you have the best conditions for falling asleep.
- Keep a dream diary – this window to your soul, to the things that are on your mind, can provide valuable insights

about what might be troubling you, and what you need to tackle in order to optimize your well-being and support being forever young.

OVER TO YOU

Now that you've read the bulk of this chapter, it's time for you to choose how exactly you are going to make the secrets of good resting *your own* by integrating them into your daily life. So...

- Close the book and consider the ways in which you would feel most able and happy to start putting this chapter's suggestions, or any other resting-related ideas of your own that you have, into practice.
- Then take a pen and notebook or piece of paper and write down the three, or five, of these ways that you most like the idea of really committing to, and that you feel will not only be really useful for you, but also achievable and sustainable. For example, you might decide to schedule in around 15 minutes somewhere in your day to meditate, or have a power nap; or you might commit to visualizing yourself every night as you go to bed waking up energized the next morning.
- If the thought of three or five things overwhelms you, just start with one – baby steps are the best way to go and as long as you keep up what you have started you'll soon find momentum building and you will want to, and be able to, do more.
- If you need a little help and encouragement to get into this decision-making zone, try the "Lost in Music" technique on page xxi to set you on your way.
- Then read your chosen action points out loud to yourself – and make an inward commitment about how, when and

where you're going to start putting them into practice – as of this week, or even *today* if possible. Feel free to write these practical details beneath the action points if you feel it will help you stick at them…

- Now use this list as your personal guide to enhancing the "Rest" section of your life-balance wheel, coming back to the list any time you feel the need to revise it or add to it…

✎

WHERE ARE YOU NOW? (PART 2)

Once you have been using the above list of action points for about a month, it will be time to assess how things are going. So – remember that list of statements you rated at the start of the chapter? Well, read and rate them again (I've listed them below, so that you don't have to flick back).

Please score the following questions for resting on a scale of 1 to 10, with 1 being "not at all true for me" and 10 being "completely true for me".

- I wake up everyday feeling rested and ready for the day ahead.
- I rarely have energy dips. My energy levels remain constant all day.
- I fall asleep easily when I go to bed and wake up energized.
- I take regular "time out" from my daily life to really rest and recuperate, such as an hour a week, or two or three weekends a year.
- I use meditation, visualization or other relaxation methods every day as a means to rest and still my mind.

Your ultimate aim in terms of a score is 40 or above – an 80 percent plus result that shows you have this secret nailed and are really using it to help you live forever young. Keep pushing yourself, however, and do what you can to avoid being complacent and slipping back into bad habits.

If you're implementing the takeaways and practising your chosen action points/techniques, I hope you'll see that your score has improved since the first time you did it.

If you're not quite where you want to be, return to the "Over to you" section in order to revisit your key action points and ensure that they still feel relevant to you (see page xx for more advice on revisiting and reassessing your goals).

After you have been practising your new "Rest" techniques for a while, don't forget to revisit your life-balance wheel at some stage (see page xxii) to keep track of progress in terms of how you feel in this area of your life. This will help you to acknowledge your achievements and to keep making further progress. The more you shade in every segment, the bigger the steps you are making along your path of living forever young!

SECRET 5: LOVE

Love, in all its beauty, holds the power to unite and divide, to bring confidence and despair, to remind us of the importance of human connection and of the ache of isolation. We both send love out into the world and attract it to us, but the most fundamental, the most crucial and influential type of love is the love we feel for ourselves. They say that love conquers all.

True love is love without judgement; it is kind, forgiving, enveloping and honest. When you can be all those things to yourself, as well as to others around you, you have unmasked the fifth secret to living forever young. Love is the essence of who we are, love is what changes the game, it's where the power is, the truth is, and to live in this place is to become unshakeable.

When our relationships with each other and with ourselves are enriching and fulfilling, our lives are nurtured with a sense of calm. Think of all the destructive feelings of love gone sour – jealousy, pride, doubt, anger, bitterness. Just saying those words, how do you feel? If you're like me, they tense you up, make you screw up your face and tighten your chest and shoulders. Now say some of the words we associate with love – forgiveness, excitement, joy, open-heartedness, kindness. For me, just thinking about those words makes me stand tall, release tension in my face and smile. My breathing feels calmer, and my attitude more positive. And these are all fundamentals for living forever young.

In this chapter we'll look at love in all its forms and in particular explore its links with forgiveness. But, before you begin, let's look at where you are with love right now.

WHERE ARE YOU NOW? PART 1

Please score the following questions for loving on a scale of 1 to 10, with 1 being "not at all true for me" and 10 being "completely true for me". Note down your score. Then, when you've completed this chapter and implemented my advice, try the questions again.

- I consciously strive to create an environment filled with love every day.
- I treat myself kindly at all times and forgive myself easily when I get things wrong or make mistakes.
- I forgive others easily when I feel hurt by them, and am able to move on with my life and my relationships.
- I am able to embrace all that life presents to me with love and appreciation.
- I feel compassion towards others who have different views to my own.

THE NEED FOR LOVE

When we talk about love and relationships, we often focus on our relationship with the significant other in our life – perhaps a wife, husband or partner. However, what if that significant other were ourselves? Self-love – the ability to show compassion, kindness and forgiveness to ourselves – is the beginning of all love, of all relationships. Because, if we can't show ourselves love, how can we expect to truly understand how to love others or invite their love into our lives?

The way in which we experience ourselves and relate to others influences all our experience of life – from the joy we

may feel for getting up in the morning, to how successful we
are at work, to how connected to others we are socially. We
wear our life's experience not only in our hearts, but in our
faces and bodies as well. Think about the subtle flickers of
emotion that pass across people's faces in response to a kind or
harsh word, or the retelling of an event. When we interact with
others, and with ourselves, our experience of those interactions
leaves its mark on our physical – and mental – well-being.
For example, think of a time when someone has offered you a
loving gesture and in doing so has made your heart sing, your
shoulders relax and your brain buzz with pride or excitement.
It's as if all the cells in your body respond to the actions and
gestures of others.

There's scientific reason for all this. The scientific study
of epigenetics considers how our environment – which doesn't
just mean our living space, but also our lifestyle and experiences
– leaves an imprint on our body's cells. So, for example, the
food you eat, the amount of exercise you do, whether you drink
alcohol or smoke, and so on, all leave their mark on our cells
through tiny genetic expressions – little notches on your genes.
These expressions can be passed from one generation to the next,
altering our DNA for our children and grandchildren. But it's
not just things we have around, or put into, our body that can
affect our cells – our stress levels, levels of relative happiness
and our sense of peace are all factors that can influence cellular
change, too. So if you think that loving yourself, being loved
and loving others is just something that has repercussions for
your emotions, think again. Love can affect change in the very
minutest of ways in your body.

Another way to look at this would be to think of it in
terms of vibrational energy. When you are in a state of anger,
for example, your cells vibrate angrily, leaving a deep and angry
energetic imprint in your body. On the other hand, when you
feel love and positivity, your cells vibrate calmly and in harmony,

like a beautiful, perfectly synchronized dance or symphony. Nurturing that synchronicity is a way to protect your cells to help you live forever young.

START WITH YOURSELF

The greatest advice I can give you about bringing more love into your life is to start with self-love. Not to be confused with selfishness or self-obsession, self-love is not arrogance or superiority or narcissism – simply put, it is the belief that you are worthy of the kind of love that you would like to share with others. Self-love is a pure acceptance and appreciation for all the parts of yourself – even the parts that you might wish to hide, whether physical, emotional or psychological.

If that sounds unrealistic, consider that this is just the beginning of your journey towards inviting more love into your life. Think of it this way: how can you accept love from someone else if you don't believe you are worthy of love yourself? Love is truly contagious. If you can love your personality, your actions, your goals and your body, you will tell the world that you are something that is worth loving. Wow. That's a lot of love. In the words of the late US actress Lucille Ball, "Love yourself first and everything falls into line."

When I ask people to describe what it means to feel love, I get the overriding sense that in general we tend to think of love as an instinctual, primal feeling that takes us by surprise, or even creeps up on us unknowingly. But, in fact, I believe that whether or not to love is simply a matter of choice – and that choice is never more relevant than when we're choosing whether or not to love ourselves. So, if self-love is a choice, how do we make that choice? And why does it often feel harder to offer it to ourselves?

Speak kindly

If a friend asks you whether or not he or she looks good in a particular outfit, what do you do? If you believe that they look great, you say so. If you think that they might look better in something else, you might say so – but in such a way as not to hurt their feelings. When you look at yourself in the mirror in an outfit you're not sure about, what do you say to yourself? Think about this for a minute. Imagine going to the mirror now... what do you see and so what do you say? If you're like the old me, you might say "Man! You look rubbish in that. Take it off. But goodness knows what else you're going to wear, because looking like that, I can't see that anything is going to look great on you." Cue wardrobe crisis – nothing is going to look great on you, because you don't believe you can look great.

What, though, if you spoke to yourself in words more like the words you'd use for a friend: "I think another colour might suit your skin-tone better", or "If it were a bit nipped at the waist, it would flatter you more."

Let's get off appearances and think about actions. If a friend makes a mistake, even if it's a big one, what are you most likely to do: forgive them and move on (you love them; if you don't move on you are basically saying you want to remove them from your life), or hit the roof and terminate the friendship forever? My guess is that most of us will offer kind words of solace and forgiveness. But would you do the same for yourself?

Often, we don't even hear how unkind we are to ourselves. We may barely recognize those negative words; we just get a pervading sense of feeling pretty rubbish. It's only when you sit and analyze how you talk to yourself that you really start to think about how unkind to yourself you can be.

So, do you think that this has a direct affect on how you age? Of course it does! When something sits unloved and uncared for, it first gets a bit dusty and stiff. Then, it might start to shrivel and wither. It doesn't see the light of day, because it's not cared for enough to make it into the light. Remember, your cells have a genetic imprint that is affected by the way you live. Live in the light – love yourself in the light – and your cells will start to vibrate in harmony.

Of course, my saying that you should ditch the negative self-talk is all well and good, but how do we go about it? For me, it's about replacing one habit (the negative habit that sees you berate yourself all the time) for another (a positive one that treats yourself with kindness). At the start you might need to do this consciously, stopping yourself as you hear the negative self-talk start. Eventually, though, with practice, you should find that positive self-talk becomes as natural as the kindness you show those around you whom you love best. Here's a step-by-step process to get you started.

- Before you begin, spend a day getting to know the voice in your head. Be really mindful of your thoughts – don't attempt to change them, just watch every one without judgement as it comes and goes across the screen of your mind. It can feel a bit odd to be "in your head" in this way, but I promise you that it will help you going forward.
- Now for the real challenge: every day watch your thoughts – only now, once you've got used to noticing them, you are going to label each one as to whether or not it serves you. Of course, some thoughts might simply be a reflection of what's going on, but when you come to a thought relating to yourself, really notice it, and ask yourself how does this thought make me feel? How does it enrich my life?
- If the answer is that it makes you feel good (perhaps through a sense of lightness in your tummy, or a sense of losing tension in your face) and it shows you how great you are in a particular way, brilliant. Bank it. You can keep it. If, though, you find it makes you scrunch up your muscles, frown or

feel anxious – if, under scrutiny, you can see no good that can come of it – ask yourself: what exactly are you criticizing about yourself?

- Now, challenge that criticism. But beware, because the quality of your challenge will determine the quality of its success. For example, if you challenge using a negative question, such as "Why am I not good enough?" or "Why don't people like me?" your brain will come up with negative answers that appear to justify every negative thing you've been telling yourself. So, instead, stop the criticism in its tracks, then ask the positive question: "Why AM I good enough?" or "Why DO people love me?"
- For each flipped question that you ask yourself, write down three reasons or positive responses. For example, if "Why am I good enough?" is your positive question, you might note down, "Because I cook supper for my family every night. Because I always arrive for meetings on time, contribute and listen carefully. Because I look after my body by running three times a week."

If you're somewhere where writing down the answers to your questions is a bit impractical, just answer them in your head. The most important thing is to stop the negative self-talk and remind yourself why it isn't valid for you and in relation to your life.

Self-love attracts love

The laws of attraction, according to US author and speaker Esther Hicks, tell us that the energy and vibrations of the messages we send out into the world about ourselves determine the ways in which other people and the world around us respond. So when you are feeling love for yourself, the universe will return positive experiences to you. I would even go so far as to say that even if you follow all other nine secrets of living

Try it now: Love yourself*

If you find it difficult to think in terms of "loving yourself", try using this affirmation to drown out the negative voice inside your head. If you like, type it out, print it and put it up all over your house so that you can see it wherever you go. Stop to read it at least once a day.

There is no one in the world the same as me. I am exactly where I am supposed to be in all moments of time. I fully and completely love, accept and embrace every part of who I am. Even the parts of me that I feel are not worthy and I would rather change, or that I feel are not serving me or my goals right now, I send them gratitude, because to deny them is to deny an aspect of myself. I fully own them as part of where I am right now in my journey and part of what makes me uniquely me. I am grateful for the lessons I learn from seeing these parts of myself and how they guide me, by showing me what I do or do not want in my life. I respond to these lessons by taking action to make change in my life and I know that every decision I make takes me closer to wholeness and complete forgiveness and acceptance in pure love.

forever young, you won't see any big changes in your overall health and well-being, or your youthfulness, if you don't make a conscious decision to love yourself. Basically, it's all about energy. The more you send out the positive, loving vibes that come from loving yourself, the more you will attract positive energy – love – back at you.

I'll give you a simple example. Think of a time when you've offered a friend a really well-intentioned, heartfelt compliment (something like, "That dress looks amazing on you!" or "I don't know what I would do without your kindness in my life – thank you") only for the friend (without any intention to dismiss you) to bat back the compliment with a comment such as, "No, I look horrible in it, but I couldn't find anything else" or "You'd probably have more fun without me!" You might feel pretty deflated and sad that your friend hadn't felt buoyed up by your compliment. His or her negative self-talk would be reflected right back at you.

Now think about how you'd feel if he or she took the compliment with a cheery smile, a thank you and perhaps a hug of gratitude – if it were me, that would make me feel good, too. And what if you were on the receiving end of the compliment? Would you accept it as intended? Or, would you have all the negative self-talk going on in the background telling you that your friend's compliment was empty and untrue?

Can you see how self-love will alter your perceptions? If you were self-loving, you would believe those lovely things about yourself, and send that love and joy right back out there.

Interestingly, I have found that when my clients start to adopt self-loving practices and mindsets, and let go of their negativity towards themselves, they more naturally begin to make life choices that support their health and well-being, rather than undermine it. US naturopath Deborah Caldwell says the same: "When women start looking at themselves through the lens of self-love, they naturally gravitate towards healthy choices, they have less desire to choose self-destructive thoughts or habits, and they feel better in both their body and mind." In my experience, it's not just women who respond like this, but men, too.

It's a true story

When one of my celebrity clients, who is now a dear friend, came to the retreat in Spain, his divorce papers were being drawn up at home – his marriage, as far as he and his wife were concerned, was over; she had lost the man she'd thought she'd married.

While he was on the retreat, though, something happened. Through our work together, getting him balanced, he was able to connect to a deeper love for himself. This changed his filter on how he was experiencing life, and there was a noticeable difference in his demeanour and attitude – his light shone and he was exuding love. He didn't want to discuss his marriage, he focused on himself and he went from being a victim to becoming a victor.

When he got home his wife was leaving. She saw him and fell to her knees. She didn't know how, but somehow she realized that the man she married had just walked back through the door. She felt his unshakable love, every wall she'd put up against the man he'd become fell down and she felt herself open-hearted and radiant. He had found pure love for himself, he shone pure love from himself, and that love came right back at him. They cancelled their divorce and are now back crazy in love, just like when they first met!

FORGIVE YOURSELF

Forgiveness expert Dr Guy Pettit, from New Zealand, says, "The forgiveness process is simply the cancellation of all the conditions in the mind that are blocking the flow of love and life energy, independently of the behaviour of others."

It can help to understand this if you think of negative emotions that block the flow of love – emotions such as guilt, anger, jealousy, all of which you need to be able to release if you are to forgive yourself and allow love to flow freely through and beyond you. There is a physical effect here, too. Studies on forgiveness have led scientists to suspect that those who have difficulty forgiving are more likely to experience heart attacks, high blood pressure, depression and other ills. Holding guilt or resentment towards yourself in any way is an act of anger. And anger over any extended period of time will put your body into fight-or-flight mode, adversely affecting your heart rate, immune response and blood pressure.

An emotional response triggers the release of certain hormones and other neurochemicals that circulate through your body to give you the physical feeling of that emotion. For example, anger or jealousy releases stress hormones (including cortisol and adrenaline) that have the effect of tensing up your muscles. In an ideal world, you'd disperse those chemicals by doing something physical – going for a run, a bike ride or a swim, say. However, emotions that have no obvious physical outlet can trigger a chain reaction that has seriously negative consequences for your well-being: they increase your heart rate, then your blood pressure. This, in turn, disrupts your digestion, and cholesterol gets dumped into your bloodstream. You'll even experience a reduced ability to think straight. Then, every time you remember what you did and cringe, those bad feelings give you a fresh hit of that chain reaction all over again.

When psychologist Charlotte van Oyen Witvliet conducted a study about forgiveness, she asked people to recall a situation whereby they believed that someone had done wrong by them. As they spent time in this memory, she monitored their physical symptoms – their bodies showed extreme signs of stress, our biggest opponent to longevity. When she asked her participants to imagine forgiving this transgression, their bodies showed signs of calming and normal responses. The same stress relief is felt when we forgive ourselves for things, too. A great weight is lifted when we truly let go and this helps to give us the freedom we deserve. Without it, we hold onto unnecessary things that don't serve us and contribute to ageing us faster. It is not always easy, but learning to forgive yourself is a vital skill in the quest for self-love, and so the quest for longevity.

Think about ways in which you beat yourself up for actions or attitudes that you have had in the past. If you feel guilty about something you've done, tell yourself that guilt is the greatest waste of time – what's done is done. You cannot change the past. Instead, think about how you could have acted differently, think about what you've learned from the situation, how your decisions can change and direct your future from now on. Consider the ways in which you've tried to make amends – whatever the outcome, you've done your best to resolve things and learned how to avoid the same mistake again. Now, let the guilt go and offer yourself forgiveness.

You can do this in a practical sense, if you like. There are many alternatives here. You might write a letter of apology to the prior situation, followed by a letter of forgiveness to yourself. You might write everything down that happened and then tear it up and burn it. Or you might try a forgiveness exercise, such as the one below.

Try it now: Ho'oponopono*

The ancient Hawaiian practice of reconciliation and forgiveness, known as ho'oponopono centres around the concept of self-responsibility for all that is. It suggests that through healing yourself (through forgiving yourself), you can heal others and the world around you. Here's how you do it:

»

- Think of something that bothers you – a personal experience that you may dwell on and find impossible to let go, but that doesn't serve you. It could be an unnecessarily sharp word to a friend, a miscommunication that got someone else into trouble, a fight you picked with a loved one because you were feeling under pressure or other areas of your life.
- Allow the feelings that your memory of that experience creates to engulf you, then take a deep breath in, and breathe out very, very slowly – as you breathe out, visualize yourself expelling all that negative energy.
- Now, either out loud or in your head, repeat the words "I forgive myself." You may want to set a timer for this, because I want you to keep repeating those simple words for a full minute.
- Then, repeat the words "Thank you" – you're thanking yourself for the forgiveness you're sharing. Express your gratitude until you feel it through your body – it may take another minute, or it may take longer. Just keep saying "Thank you" until you can feel that gratitude resonate through every cell in your body.
- Now say to yourself "I love you." Really feel the love – keep repeating it until you feel completely enveloped in gentle, nurturing self-love.

How does that feel to you? What does your body feel like immediately after completing the exercise? Do you feel like you have released something? Do you feel lighter in any way?

SHARING LOVE

Now the we've looked at how to love ourselves better, we can start to think about how to share that love with others and the world around us, in turn bringing yet more love into our own lives.

It's interesting to know that many studies have shown that people in long-term, supportive and healthy relationships live longer. In a study conducted by Harvard University in 2013, researchers found that married people were more likely to detect cancers in their bodies earlier, as well as more likely to recover, than those who were not married. Additional studies have shown that men who have never married are three times more likely to die of a heart attack than those who have a wife. While all of this may seem to be making a case for marriage, rather than love, one of the deciding factors inherent in this Western cultural phenomena is that the act of marriage is representative of connected and healthy relationships and a secure emotional support system. Positive social interaction is the key – isolation and loneliness take a terrible toll on our well-being and are top factors for a lowered life expectancy. The good news is that the opposite – loving relationships of all kinds – are a vital component in our living forever young.

Now that you've made the decision to love yourself – warts and all – let's think about what happens when we share the love we feel with others and love them, too. I need to make this clear as its not just about being *in* love, but about loving yourself and all others with whom you have a relationship – friends and family, as well as partners.

Let's look at how to bring more love into our lives with each of those groups of people.

Loving friendships

The nature of friendship is complex, intriguing and potentially so, so rewarding. Humans are sociable beings, and we need connection with a "pack" in order to thrive. If you think back to our distant, primitive ancestors, those who formed groups to support each other, protect each other and gather food to share with the community were those who survived.

While some friendships are instant, others require a bit of nurturing and skill to develop – but all good friendships deserve your time and commitment. I recently read a newspaper article about someone whose close friend had died. During the early weeks of her grief, she received dozens of messages from mutual friends from their past expressing sadness and condolences. The messages got her thinking – these were people who'd been lost from her life and the life of her friend, but who now wanted to share in her very personal, very private grief. It made her realize just how precious, how deep and how meaningful true friendship really is.

Now, I'm not suggesting that you need to start investing hours of your time in every social media "friend" you have going. Instead, think of those four, maybe five, people in your life who are unrelated to you, but whose presence enriches you every day, every week – even if you're not with them. Invest time in those friendships, offer simple acts of gratitude and kindness (by way of a call, a written note, a small gift sent through the post). Cherish these friendships, they are precious. The good feelings you get from giving to, and receiving from, such friends provides a well-being boost that is a key ingredient for so many of the secrets to living forever young.

Loving partnerships

In a loving, productive relationship you only have to think of that person and you light up instantly and start glowing. Every morning when I wake, I always share three things that I'm grateful for with my partner. It might be: "I'm grateful for how we laughed yesterday", "I'm grateful for the dinner you prepared for us yesterday" and "I'm grateful for how you told me you believed in me when things didn't go to plan." Sharing three different statements about something tangible that happened the day before pulls us together and reminds us how much we appreciate and respect one another in our daily lives; how every day together matters and enriches us.

If you are in a relationship, try sharing three things with your partner each day – with the wonders of technology you can do this even when you aren't physically together – and notice how positively it affects your whole day and how it unfolds.

Loving family

Your family was the first experience you ever had of love. Whether that family is natural, blended or adoptive, our connection to those we grow up with is unbreakable – even if we move away, or even if we find ourselves deep in family feud. The simple fact of the matter is that shared life experience connects us in ways that are impossible to replicate in any other relationship.

I value my family above all else and I make my family my priority. I have plenty of friends whose relationship with their family is more tricky – where difficult dynamics make it hard to feel close. But ask yourself this: when the chips are down, who would have your back? For most of us, it's our family.

That's not to say, however, that there aren't relationships within families that take on a destructive force. In those cases, as with any negativity in your life, you have to find your power and your love and remove yourself to a place of safety and light. And you have to do so without guilt. Remember you can only be responsible for your own life and actions, and not those of anyone else.

Unless you fall into this category, try practising gratitude for your family as well. Think of three things that you are grateful for in relation to your family or a specific family member. Tell them, if you can, or just say them aloud or to yourself. The very act of identifying and naming the three things will have dramatic effects. You'll be surprised – our fuse is usually so short with our family and a part of you may really not want to do it, but you will only evolve if you do. Lay down your weapons of war and roll up your sleeves, reopen up your heart and get on with it, with love!

Stress causes the aging process. Attitude is what keeps a person young, that's what keeps them healthy. That's what stimulates them to creativity and to be happy.

Burt Goldman –
"The American Monk", meditation master

THE HUG FIX

Hugs and physical touch are an amazing way to share love, kindness and forgiveness. Studies have shown that ten hugs a day can help us to thrive. But you can start with just one. This whole process is about *your* next step, and once you take a step you can build on it ad infinitum. Embracing others with a genuine hug where you give and receive love at the same time builds trust and boosts levels of the hormone oxytocin (otherwise known as the "love hormone"). This plays an essential role in human bonding – for example, it's also the hormone that floods the mother's system as she comforts and nurses her baby. Interestingly, studies have shown that oxytocin can block the sensation of emotional or physical pain, giving the body a brief respite that enables it to start healing itself, even physically. To use the mother and baby example again – it's thought that it's that first rush of oxytocin high as a new mother holds her baby that might be a significant contributing factor to the way in which she forgets the pain of labour and childbirth.

Furthermore, a prolonged hug will stimulate the body to increase serotonin levels – serotonin is the hormone that boosts mood and makes us feel good. Hugging may also stimulate the action of the thymus gland, which in turn helps build up the immune system. It builds presence, by encouraging you to stop activity and connect, which also increases your general sense of well-being and belonging in the world. It also helps you to feel safe and secure and helps to calm your parasympathetic nervous system. There are so many ways in which a good embrace can lift the sense of wellness within our human bodies.

And what happens when our bodies feel good? That's right… they are healthier and they live longer.

FORGIVING OTHERS

In the same way that you need to forgive yourself in order to reap rewards in your physical and mental health, you also need to learn to forgive others. Without forgiving those who have wronged you, you filter experience through the negative lens of holding onto experiences and emotions that would be better let go.

Of course, it's not always easy to forgive. And sometimes, it will feel not appropriate. This is where you need to learn how powerful forgiveness is and how it gives you freedom, and makes you a better person, even when it feels the least natural thing in the world to do. I'm not suggesting that every person you forgive necessarily needs a place back in your life; just that in order to make sure you have only love in your life, you have to let go of your anger and resentment towards others, just as you have to let go of anger towards yourself. Here's an exercise to help you open yourself up to the notion of forgiving others.

• Acknowledge the wrongdoing – what is it that you need to forgive? Why? How does it make you feel? Why did it hurt you? Who is it that you hold responsible for making you feel this way? Write that person's name down in the middle of a piece of paper and draw a circle around it. (If there's more than one person, write all their names in the circle.)

- Now, around the circle (turn the paper as you go) write the statement "I value health, love and joy more than disease. I want to live a long, happy, healthy and fulfilled life."

- Divide the whole piece of paper into four by drawing a line down and a line across the page, stopping and starting around the words you've written and the encircled name(s). At the top of one of the four spaces write the word Problem, in another write Emotions, in another write Values, and in the final quarter write the word Release.

- In the first quarter, write a brief description of what happened – just a single word or sentence will do. Be really succinct! In the second, write three overriding emotions that you felt when it happened (sadness, anger, jealously, for example). In the third, identify the values that you hold that you feel have been compromised or overridden through the problem. (Those values are important, because the fact that you have them means you have a source of dignity and power.) You don't need to write anything in the final quarter – because release is an empty, free space that can be filled again with love, which is where you're heading.

- Look at the blank space. Whatever you have wished for in the past for the person who has upset you, imagine sending it into that space and watching it disappear. Forget it, let it go – completely, if you can. Imagine it shrinking to a dot and disappearing. In doing so, you release your negative emotions (the emotions that are blocking the flow of love and good vibes in your system) and you give back responsibility to the other person. By doing this, you'll become free.

LOVING YOUR WORLD

Think of all the great sights your eyes have given you. Remember that you hear music and a bird singing without even trying. Think of the amazing memories your brain allows you to recall at will. Realize that your immune system is there to protect and repair you without you thinking about it. Be grateful for all the gifts (whether material, emotional or physical) that bring joy into your life.

Too many of us live our lives in regret, disappointment and dissatisfaction. Yet we are living longer, with more material assets and more reason to be grateful for life than any humans since the beginning of time.

Think of all the reasons your world gives you to experience love – love of yourself, of people around you, of your environment, of your life. We'll talk more later on about how to feel gratitude and how to appreciate your inner and outer environments, so for now just let yourself feel love for your world and the blessings it gives. Think how much sunnier and more positive the world seems when you send love out into it because you've learned to be open to this power no matter what happens in life. You can be your best.

Tomorrow, try a little game with yourself. Take the opportunity to tell every person you interact with what you love – or at least really like – about them. You don't have to be too deep and meaningful. This is really just about getting used to the notion of using the word "love" and so feeling the emotion. When you buy something from a shop, tell the checkout operator that you love the colour of the top he or she is wearing; tell the guy on the coffee stand that you love his coffee better than any other; tell your colleague that you love what they've done with their hair, or that piece of work they submitted last week. But make sure your comments are genuine. If they're fake, you'll feel it (and so will the person on the receiving end). Make sure you feel the love as you give it. What happens each time you use the word "love" in those interactions? My guess is you'll be treated by a beaming smile and a heartfelt thank you, and feel a bit of love right back.

NOW YOU CAN LOVE

No matter what you do, aim to do it with love. Through the pain, the rejections, the abuse, the challenges there is only one thing more powerful than negativity: an unshakeable connection to love. Love is within you and it will not only give you strength and courage, but also freedom. Your life is worth every drop of effort that you're prepared to give it, but it won't even feel like effort if every ounce of your commitment is layered with love. When you're in love with how you live, it's there that you'll find your peace. Love will become your fuel and keep you going, give you resilience and commitment, when most would have given up. People tell me that I have energy in abundance, but it's love that fuels that energy. In the midst of the maelstrom of life, voices of doubt, fear and regret are silenced only by a voice filled with love.

LIVING FOREVER YOUNG
TOP 10 TAKEAWAYS: LOVE

- Consider how the love you feel for life now will leave an imprint on your cells to be passed to future generations of your family – your love matters.
- Love yourself before attempting to love anyone else.
- Switch negative self-talk to positive self-talk – be kind to yourself, just as you hope other people would be kind to you.

- Forgive yourself, always. You're human. You make mistakes. Learn from them, apologize for them if you need to, but then move on.
- Remember that your response to situations will attract similar in return – love and be loved.
- Share your love – tell your family you love them (often), show loving kindness to your friends, treat acquaintances with respect, honour those who are kind to you, be polite in all your interactions (even with people you don't personally know).
- Don't shy away from physical affection – a hug has a physiological response in your body and floods you with love!
- Forgive other people when they have upset you in some way – holding onto your anger or resentment means that you've reduced the space within you for love. It doesn't serve you – let it go.
- Love the world around you because it's precious and it nurtures and sustains you.
- Fuel your energy with love. With the power of love in everything you do, you're unstoppable.

OVER TO YOU

Now that you've read the bulk of this chapter, it's time for you to choose how exactly you are going to make the secrets of good loving *your own* by integrating them into your daily life. So…

- Close the book and consider the ways in which you would feel most able and happy to start putting this chapter's suggestions, or any other loving-related ideas of your own that you have, into practice.

- Then take a pen and notebook or piece of paper and write down the three, or five, of these ways that you most like the idea of really committing to, and that you feel will not only be really useful for you, but also achievable and sustainable. For example, you might commit to finding and acknowledging something you love about the people you come into connection with – maybe over the course of a week or even just a day; look at yourself in a mirror and recognize something you truly love about yourself, however small or silly it may seem; or ask those close to you to tell you something that they love about you.
- If the thought of three or five things overwhelms you, just start with one – baby steps are the best way to go and as long as you keep up what you have started you'll soon find momentum building and you will want to, and be able to, do more.
- If you need a little help and encouragement to get into this decision-making zone, try the "Lost in Music" technique on page xxi to set you on your way.
- Then read your chosen action points out loud to yourself – and make an inward commitment about how, when and where you're going to start putting them into practice – as of this week, or even *today* if possible. Feel free to write these practical details beneath the action points if you feel it will help you stick at them…
- Now use this list as your personal guide to enhancing the "Love" section of your life-balance wheel, coming back to the list any time you feel the need to revise it or add to it…

WHERE ARE YOU NOW? (PART 2)

Once you have been using the above list of action points for about a month, it will be time to assess how things are going. So – remember that list of statements you rated at the start of the chapter? Well, read and rate them again (I've listed them below, so that you don't have to flick back).

Please score the following questions for loving on a scale of 1 to 10, with 1 being "not at all true for me" and 10 being "completely true for me".

- I consciously strive to create an environment filled with love every day.
- I treat myself kindly at all times and forgive myself easily when I get things wrong or make mistakes.
- I forgive others easily when I feel hurt by them, and am able to move on with my life and my relationships.
- I am able to embrace all that life presents to me with love and appreciation.
- I feel compassion towards others who have different views to my own.

Your ultimate aim in terms of a score is 40 or above – an 80 percent plus result that shows you have this secret nailed and are really using it to help you live forever young. Keep pushing yourself, however, and do what you can to avoid being complacent and slipping back into bad habits.

If you're implementing the takeaways and practising your chosen action points/techniques, I hope you'll see that your score has improved since the first time you did it.

If you're not quite where you want to be, return to the "Over to you" section in order to revisit your key action points and ensure that they still feel relevant to you (see page xx for more advice on revisiting and reassessing your goals).

After you have been practising your new "Love" techniques for a while, don't forget to revisit your life-balance wheel at some stage (see page xxii) to keep track of progress in terms of how you feel in this area of your life. This will help you to acknowledge your achievements and to keep making further progress. The more you shade in every segment, the bigger the steps you are making along your path of living forever young!

SECRET 6: SHINE

I don't think I know a single person who doesn't feel better when the sun comes out – myself included. Sunlight immediately makes me feel more active, energetic, balanced and strengthened, and less nervous. Sunny days feel longer and, over the course of the year, the sun shows glorious yellows, oranges and reds – warm colours that help reflect our inner glow. The sun is a symbol of positivity and energy.

In this chapter we'll look at the nature of "Shine" in two ways. First, at how the shining light of the sun is essential to your physical and mental well-being (it even helps to manufacture vital vitamin D). And, second, at how the notion of shining provides a metaphor for your own radiance, so that you can shine your own light into your life and into the lives of others. I'll show you how you can always shine no matter what the challenge. Like the sun, shining your light in the world is a selfless and yet nourishing act – giving and never asking for anything back. Your light is the seed of all life and creativity. And we'll look at how to find and harness the light that shines from those around you.

But, before we begin, let's look at where you are with the concepts of shining and being shone upon right now.

✎

WHERE ARE YOU NOW? (PART 1)

Please score the following questions for shining on a scale of 1 to 10, with 1 being "not at all true for me" and 10 being "completely true for me". Note down your score. Then, when you've completed this chapter and implemented its advice, try the questions again.

- I feel more positive when I'm outside in the sunshine.
- I understand the all-giving power of the sun and its importance for sustaining life on Earth.
- I feel light radiate within me in the form of a positive outlook on life.
- I try to shine light into the lives of others every day.
- I use the sun as a focus for meditation.

THE NEED TO BE SHONE UPON

Many people I talk to identify with the feelings of low mood, sadness and even depression that come with the times of year where the sun is low in the sky, the days are short, and the darkness lingers. There's even a name for that condition – Seasonal Affective Disorder (SAD). Its symptoms are fatigue, lowered motivation, sleepiness, increased appetite, weight gain, irritability and decreased sociability. So why is sunlight so important for your health, and in particular for helping you to feel and look younger for longer?

A study conducted by Karolinska University Hospital and Lund University in Sweden, which followed the sunlight behaviour of 29,518 women for 20 years, has demonstrated that women who stay out of the sun live 0.6 to 2.1 years less than women who sunbathe regularly. It appears that moderate sun exposure can actually decrease the risk of heart disease and other non-cancer-related diseases – although we don't yet fully understand why. Dr Pelle Lindqvist, who ran the study, has said that avoiding the sun could have the same effect on your life expectancy as smoking: "We found smokers in the highest sun exposure group were at a similar risk as non-smokers who avoided sun exposure, indicating avoidance of sun exposure to be a risk factor of the same magnitude as smoking." While this sounds quite controversial, we should remember that there is no life on our planet without the sun. It is our energy source and avoiding it can create problems whereas exposing ourselves to it (in safe measure) fuels us up with its goodness. The happy, healthy glow that many of us have after a holiday in the sun is testament to this.

THE CIRCADIAN RHYTHM

Everything in nature has a daily rhythm. It exists in all living things – from the cells in a blade of grass to the cells in your body. We call it our circadian rhythm (see page 86), and although it is largely a biological process, external factors such as light and temperature can influence its function. For example, if you travel across time zones, as I often do, the best way to combat jet lag is to use sunlight to reset your circadian rhythm to local time – whatever time you get to bed, make sure you get up to get out into the morning light. This will tell your brain which time zone you're in and will speed up the process of readjustment.

In this sense, then, light regulates us. People with regularly disrupted circadian rhythms (such as those who work shifts, or who travel long distances frequently) can be prone to SAD-type conditions at any time of year, affecting their physical and mental well-being. However, there are lots of ways in which to get your circadian rhythm on track, even if you are a shift-worker or regular traveller. Among them are eating at set mealtimes, consciously managing stress levels and following all the principles of getting a good amount of sleep (you can check those out in Secret 4: Rest). Most of all, though, enhancing your exposure to natural light – letting the sun shine on you – and getting outdoors as much as possible are the most effective and simplest ways to combat SAD symptoms and harness the well-being power of the sun.

SUNSHINE AND YOUR BODY

Having talked about the power of the sun in general terms – how it helps to regulate your body clock – let's look at some of the specific benefits there are to having the sun shine on your body.

We all know that over-exposure to the UV rays of the sun can cause skin cancer and it is vitally important that we protect ourselves against that by screening our skin against the sun. However, the sun's UV rays are also, in the correct dosage, health-giving, because they help the body to manufacture vitamin D.

Although we get most of our vitamins from our food, vitamin D is primarily manufactured in the body in response to the skin's exposure to the UV rays of the sun. In 2014, the University of Cambridge published findings from a study that found an estimated 91 percent of people living in the UK don't get enough vitamin D. That's a problem. We need vitamin D because it has been shown to help prevent memory loss and even Alzheimer's as we age, as well as being essential for the long-lasting health of our bones, because it improves the absorption of calcium from our food. This means staving off illnesses such as osteoporosis (associated with ageing in women), as well as other bone-related conditions, such as rickets. Diabetes, acne, eczema and psoriasis are all associated with lowered levels of vitamin D. Furthermore, vitamin D regulates cell growth, which some researchers have found can help prevent the formation of cancer cells.

And yet the answer is right there, up in the sky, for you every day.

In order to manufacture the right levels of vitamin D to keep you healthy, you need to go outside and expose at least 40 percent of your skin (say, your arms, face, legs and belly) to the sunlight without sunscreen (which blocks the passage of UV light into the skin) for about 20 minutes every day. On a cloudy day you might need to flash the flesh for a bit longer, but remember that the sun's rays penetrate even the darkest clouds. If you have dark skin, you would generally need more exposure than fair-skinned people; if you're a fair-skinned redhead, you'll probably need less. Older people and people with more body fat might need a bit longer. In general terms, during a 30-minute sun bath, your body produces about 20,000 IUs of vitamin D, which is as much as in 200 glasses of milk. Wow! However, if there's no cloud there's also sun danger. So, how do we balance our basic physiological need for sunlight with what we know to be harmful about the sun?

Aim for about half the time it would take you to get sunburn, but never ever push that so that you do actually burn. I recommend sunbathing for 2 minutes each on your front, back and sides, then gradually increase the time by 1 minute each day, and find out the length of time that is comfortable for you.

If you were wondering, the UV rays from ultraviolet tanning beds don't count either – you need the actual sun to shine its light on your skin for the physiological process of manufacturing vitamin D to work.

Facing the practicality

As lovely as it would be to think that every day is filled with sunshine, for most of us in many places in the world, it just doesn't happen. And, even when the sun is shining beautifully, we might be stuck indoors doing our jobs. What's the answer? Simple: get out as much as you can, as often as you can. Choose to eat your breakfast outdoors on a sunny day (looking through the window and turning your face to the sun doesn't count), and at the weekends or during the long, summer evenings, take yourself for a walk that keeps you outside for as long as possible (if it's very sunny, follow the usual precautions on burning; and during the summer months avoid the hottest part of the day between 11am and 3pm when the sun is at its strongest and will most likely burn you).

During the winter, wrap up and still get out – even if it's just your face and hands that are exposed, it's better than nothing at all. And, anyway, being outside in the light and air is good for your mental and spiritual health even when the sun isn't shining. Finally, during the winter months, consider a vitamin D supplement (see page 68) – just to boost your levels while sunlight is scarce.

A word of warning

One final word to be absolutely clear: I'm not advocating that you bathe in the sun without sunscreen so that you come anywhere near to burning your skin. Sunburn damages skin cells and can cause cancer. That's a fact. Always operate within safe limits of sun exposure.

SUNSHINE AND YOUR MIND

I don't know about you but I feel better when the sun is shining. And when I say better – I mean more alive, alert and positive. I feel fundamentally happier. It could be coincidence, but whenever I go to the Philippines for my live events (a place that gets on average 2,100 hours of sunlight a year, compared with about 1,450 hours in London), I really notice how much happier everyone seems. I feel a friend in almost every person I connect with in the Philippines; I feel the positivity that those who live there send out into the world. The mood is infectious and their good vibes make me feel good, too. What's fascinating is that while this positivity could be just coincidence, actually there is physiology involved in the fact that sunshine causes happiness.

The body's primary feel-good hormone is serotonin. Studies on rats show that there are greater levels of serotonin circulating in the rats' bodies when they have been exposed to natural sunlight. Interestingly, another study involving autopsies on humans after death showed that those who died after an extended period of sunny, summer days had more serotonin in their systems that those who died after a period of cloudy, dark winter days. Overall, studies show that it's sunlight (rather than temperature) that is the key.

Interestingly, serotonin is partly manufactured in your pineal gland – the gland, as small as a grain of rice and shaped like a pine cone (hence its name), which sits deep within your brain, in line with your eyes. I believe that the quality of your life comes down to the quality of the emotions that you feel every day, and this gland has a major influence on that because its secretions change according to your stress levels, your seasonal and daily circadian rhythms, and your physical performance. Sunshine activates the pineal gland to send out the hormones that make us feel good.

Again, then, the advice is obvious: when the sun shines, get out and enjoy it, turn your face to the sun and let its light shine into you, improving your mood and helping you yourself to shine.

Capturing this life-force energy from the sun is fundamental in fuelling you up with this free, yet powerful, energy that feeds all life on this planet – plants, trees, animals and, of course, human beings. The sun was here before us and will be here after us. It has something to give us that allows us to shine our light into life so that we always have the energy to do what we need on our journey in living forever young.

CULTURES OF THE SUN: SUN AND SPIRIT

The sun gives life to our planet. As a result, since time immemorial cultures the world over have believed in honouring the sun and trying to harness its power. Ancient sites such as

Stonehenge, in Wiltshire, UK, demonstrate unfathomable understanding of the movement of the sun across the heavens for our prehistoric ancestors, with massive stones and plinths positioned so that at the midsummer solstice the sun's rays are channelled precisely across the site. The ancient Greeks and Romans honoured the gods Helios and Sol, respectively. In Japanese lore, Amaterasu was both the goddess of the sun and of the universe. Pre-dynastic Egyptians honoured Atum as their sun-god and ancient Egyptians would gaze at the sun holding metal rods, to harness and amplify its powerful energy. The ancient Aztecs of Mexico made many attempts to find their perfect sun god, whose power they knew would determine survival on Earth.

The commonality between all these traditions is that the sun is life-giving energy and that's why, even today, we try to harness its power in order to raise our spirit to a higher, more positive level.

Sun "worshipping"

When I host my retreats in Spain, we watch the sun rise out of the sea and I take the participants through a sunrise meditation, followed by a Salute to the Sun yoga sequence that welcomes us to the new day and harnesses the power of the all-giving sun. Others practise sun gazing – looking at the sun for a short period of time when it just peeks above the horizon and is at its lowest in the sky.

Now, of course, we are told that we should never look straight at the sun, but just as it pops over the edge of the Earth at sunrise or dips at sunset, its wavelengths are short and the rays at their weakest. Sun gazers believe that as long as we look for only a few seconds, the practice is safe. They stand barefoot to feel a deep connection with the Earth, and look at the sun for a few seconds, before breaking away to avoid eye damage. The theory behind this is that the sun, as life-giver, can feed the body and mind with an abundance of energy. Some claim that sun-gazing has reversed the shrinkage of the pineal gland that happens naturally as we age. If this is something that interests you, do your research – it is still a controversial practise but one that I believe can bring great benefits when exercised correctly.

However, you don't need to do anything as formal as sunrise meditation, morning yoga or sun gazing to benefit from the power of the rising sun. Wherever you are, you can harness its magic, even from your bedroom window, your back garden or a hilltop in your local park. The sun fills us with power, energy and love – and in my case, those three things help me to be the best version of me. Making time to witness its power rising in whatever way possible raises the spirit and reminds us to spend our own day shining. You can even benefit from the sun though a closed window – so if this is your only option, go for it. It is always best to experience it with no filter, no clouds, nothing at all, but any sunlight is better than none. And remember, if you are going out in the sun, take things a step at a time. Some people are more sensitive than others and you should always be aware of your personal limits on this score.

SEEING THE LIGHT WITHIN YOU

I remember when I was told I was never going to walk again. I went into a very dark place. Then, I heard that Bruce Lee had broken his back and, like me, had wondered how he would ever come back from his place of darkness again. But he did – and he came back even stronger than before. I remember the specific moment I learned about that, because it felt like a light had been switched back on within me, shining some hope on the situation I was in.

That light first produced hope. Then, the more I hoped, the more I believed. As the light began to glow brighter, it came to represent the love and trust I now have for life, other people, the universe, and myself.

When you feel compassion for yourself and for others, when you live your life with belief, passion and purpose, when you make sure that you get enough rest, breathe into the spaces and look after your body and mind, when you follow all the secrets of living forever young, your light within glows brighter. You'll feel more confident and discover more freedom within your own mind. You'll also give yourself permission to play a lot more with life, because you're more conscious in each moment. All that from simply finding the light within you.

It's a true story

A participant in one of my retreats had experienced some pretty hardcore emotional challenges in her life. These left her protecting her heart and never really committing to a solid relationship, which was stopping her from shining and fulfilling her potential. She said she had been living with heart pain for over 40 years. While on the retreat I helped reconnect her to the truth and her inner strength and, as a result, she started to let go of the resistance she was holding on to. In those moments she starting shining her light again and, as she started radiating, she literally started to look younger and feel the freedom that she had been longing for. Everyone was amazed because it happened so fast and when we showed her a mirror she couldn't believe what she saw in her reflection. She glowed and shone with a new beauty and elegance that instantly lit her life back up. Within a few weeks her partner moved in and she said that by shining like the sun she felt a love she hadn't experienced ever before. I remember her sharing her story on stage and it bringing many people to tears.

Try it now: Inner light meditation*

Try out the following meditation on your inner light, which is intended to help you feel that glow within you, using the sun's energy as a metaphor. The whole practise should take you around ten minutes but there is no set amount of time for it. Practise it as often as you can.

- Sit or lie comfortably, somewhere where you'll be undisturbed. Close your eyes and inhale deeply – as you do so feel your body relax; then feel it relax some more as you let your breath out again. Take several long, deep breaths, each time feeling more at ease and more centred. Go into a deep state of restfulness where you feel calm and comfortable.
- Imagine that you are lying down in a warm, grassy meadow with the golden sun rays shining gently on you. Feel the sun rays gently hit your skin, and feel your body absorb them so that they gather within you in the middle of your chest, at your "heart centre". Be thankful for this life-giving energy as you watch it become a beautiful orb of light inside you.
- Consider the source of that light – the sun has been a source of energy for millions of years. It is the same sun that shone on the dinosaurs, the Egyptians, your ancestors, your childhood – and now it's shining on you as an adult, feeding you its life-giving energy, just as it always did.
- Feel the warmth of the glowing orb within you, spreading throughout your body, into your organs and tissues. Visualize the power, energy and »

positivity spreading through you. Imagine yourself beginning to radiate and glow with the energy.

- Consider the healing power of this energy and allow the warmth to heal you mentally, emotionally, physically and spiritually. Tune into the feeling of the energy coursing through you, growing as your healing grows and expands.

- Now imagine yourself projecting the shining light of that orb outside of you. Imagine filling the room with pure, positive healing from the light within you.

- Now imagine that light filling the whole building you are in, then the town or city, then the country. Imagine the light that has come directly from you encircling the whole world and finally going out into the whole universe. You have blessed everything with your light.

- Finally, bring to mind someone you know who needs specific healing – perhaps a friend going through a difficult separation, illness or bereavement; or a family member having a stressful time with a job. Imagine directing your light specifically into their heart, filling them with your healing power, too.

- Bring your attention back to yourself and really connect to your heart centre, knowing that this is where your light glows, it is the source of your power and energy. Let your power shine out always from this point. Remember how good it makes you feel to be filled with that positive glow, and the energy you have to transmit to the world around you.

- Take a deep breath and stretch out your legs, arms and back in any way that seems comfortable to you, gently bringing yourself back to the present.

»

> • Wiggle your fingers and toes, then open your
>   eyes. Notice how you feel – refreshed, vibrant and
>   positive. Remember to harness that energy within
>   you whenever you need it – for your own good or
>   the good of others. It's always within you and always
>   shining outwards.

**To give your life to serve, to help the planet –
to me that keeps you young forever.**
Guru Mukh – Kundalini yoga expert,
teacher and author

SEEING THE LIGHT IN OTHERS

I have had the good fortune to work very closely with some
of the world's top shamans – healers who converse with the
spirit world to effect good on Earth. Something I have noticed
about every one of them is that, despite what is potentially a
very serious business of interacting with good and evil spirits
to create powerful change in people's lives, they just don't take
life too seriously. Their manner is always lighthearted, always
shining. One of the most important lessons I've learned from
these people is always to see the light in others – in other
words, always to seek out the good in everyone I come across,
no matter how difficult or challenging that might seem to
be. In a similar way, when a yoga practitioner greets you or
leaves you with the word *namaste* (or, hands closed in prayer
and a small bow – which is the physical representation of that
word), he or she means "the light in me respects and honours
the light in you."

Seeing the light in others is, I think, one of the reasons that shamans are such positive, happy people. After all, if we treat everyone as if they have something positive to offer our relationship and the world, we approach them with an open-heartedness that is reflected back at us (we learned this in Secret 5: Love). Even those who hurt us, or set out purposely to wrongfoot us have a light within. Set yourself a challenge for today (and then extend it to every day, if you can). Make a conscious effort not to see the bad or irritating in people. Instead, greet and treat everyone you meet the same, looking only for the positives. For example, instead of approaching your boss with the attitude that he or she is grumpy all the time, remind yourself of the wisdom he or she has to share with you, and start your interaction with that in mind. Instead of meeting a tricky colleague who tries to undermine you with resentment, approach them confidently and suggest how you could collaborate using your ideas for a particular project as well as their own (remember, flattering your colleague's efforts – and believing their worth – will make them more open to receiving your ideas, too).

It's harder than you think to be positive with everyone you meet. As we age, we become more cynical and often suspicious of other people, especially those we don't know. It's almost as if we silently ask them to prove they are worthy of our respect and love, before they've had a chance to show it for themselves. But, what if we started out with a sense of trust – like a child does? How many more of our interactions would be positive, rather than negative or ineffectual? Even if it's only one, it's one more positive interaction than you will have had yesterday. So, go on, take up the challenge. Greet everyone with the spirit of *namaste*, and resolve to see their light. At the end of the day reflect on how doing so has made your own light glow brighter and shone light on your own life. There's no doubt that when you glow, you look better to others, you feel better within yourself, you're nicer to be around and in those moments you are living forever young.

NOW YOU CAN SHINE

At the start of this chapter we reinforced the notion that the sun is continually shining and giving life-force energy not just to you, but to every living organism on the planet. We learned to harness that power in a metaphorical sense to energize our own lives and bodies. Presenting ourselves to the world with the intention of shining our light into all our interactions makes the world itself seem more positive. However, the most important message I want to send you away with is that shining is your natural state. Once you recognize your inner glow, you won't ever need to force it or fake it – just be you and have fun lighting up places, people and situations wherever you go.

LIVING FOREVER YOUNG
TOP 10 TAKEAWAYS: SHINE

- Always resolve to shine in every situation, no matter what else is going on.
- Light is a representation of your greatness – welcome and cherish it.
- Spend time in the sunshine to manufacture vitamin D in your body – remembering the rules relating to sunburn and UV rays, too, of course.
- Have fun in the sun whenever it shines – it is proven to make you feel good.
- Act like the sun, always giving, always shining, never asking for anything in return.
- Find the light in others – even if it eludes you at first.

- Challenges in your life are opportunities for you to shine brighter than you have ever shone before.
- Watch the rising sun at least once in your life – consider its passage across the sky, one of the only constants in life.
- Use your light to send healing to someone who is suffering, emotionally, physically or spiritually.
- Feel the warmth of light, keeping you safe and secure, within you every day.

OVER TO YOU

Now that you've read the bulk of this chapter, it's time for you to choose how exactly you are going to make the secrets of shining *your own* by integrating them into your daily life. So…

- Close the book and consider the ways in which you would feel most able and happy to start putting this chapter's suggestions, or any other shining-related ideas of your own that you have, into practice.
- Then take a pen and notebook or piece of paper and write down the three, or five, of these ways that you most like the idea of really committing to, and that you feel will not only be really useful for you, but also achievable and sustainable. For example, you might commit to getting out into the sun (or at least outdoors) for 20 minutes a day; or taking a great-quality vitamin D supplement; or to sharing your own light with others by showing kindness and compassion to a loved one, or even a stranger, in need.
- If the thought of three or five things overwhelms you, just start with one – baby steps are the best way to go and as long as you keep up what you have started you'll soon find momentum building and you will want to, and be able to, do more.

- If you need a little help and encouragement to get into this decision-making zone, try the "Lost in Music" technique on page xxi to set you on your way.
- Then read your chosen action points out loud to yourself – and make an inward commitment about how, when and where you're going to start putting them into practice – as of this week, or even *today* if possible. Feel free to write these practical details beneath the action points if you feel it will help you stick at them…
- Now use this list as your personal guide to enhancing the "Shine" section of your life-balance wheel, coming back to the list any time you feel the need to revise it or add to it…

✎

WHERE ARE YOU NOW? (PART 2)

Once you have been using the above list of action points for about a month, it will be time to assess how things are going. So – remember that list of statements you rated at the start of the chapter? Well, read and rate them again (I've listed them below, so that you don't have to flick back).

Please score the following questions for shining on a scale of 1 to 10, with 1 being "not at all true for me" and 10 being "completely true for me".

- I feel more positive when I'm outside in the sunshine.
- I understand the all-giving power of the sun and its importance for sustaining life on Earth.
- I feel light radiate within me in the form of a positive outlook on life.
- I try to shine light into the lives of others every day.
- I use the sun as a focus for meditation.

Your ultimate aim in terms of a score is 40 or above – an 80 percent plus result that shows you have this secret nailed and are really using it to help you live forever young. Keep pushing yourself, however, and do what you can to avoid being complacent and slipping back into bad habits.

If you're implementing the takeaways and practising your chosen action points/techniques, I hope you'll see that your score has improved since the first time you did it.

If you're not quite where you want to be, return to the "Over to you" section in order to revisit your key action points and ensure that they still feel relevant to you (see page xx for more advice on revisiting and reassessing your goals).

After you have been practising your new "Shine" techniques for a while, revisit your life-balance wheel (see page xxii) to keep track of progress in terms of how you feel in this area of your life. This will help you to acknowledge your achievements and make further progress. The more you shade in every segment, the bigger the steps you are making to live forever young!

SECRET 7: BELIEVE

US boxer Sugar Ray Robinson once said, "To be a champ you have to believe in yourself when no one else will." I think that in order to have that self-belief, we need to live an authentic life that reflects our passions and our purpose, bringing with them a sense of fulfilment and meaning. When we tune in to the vibrations within, and are true to ourselves, self-belief follows because everything we do reflects everything we value.

In this chapter we'll look at the differences between a passion and a purpose, and you'll learn techniques that will help you identify what you believe in and what you're aiming for, so that you can move forward with the conviction that while learning how to live forever young you're also living an authentic, valuable and rewarding life.

But, before you begin, let's look at where you are with belief right now.

✎
WHERE ARE YOU NOW? (PART 1)

Please score the following questions for believing on a scale of 1 to 10, with 1 being "not at all true for me" and 10 being "completely true for me". Note down your score. Then when you've completed this chapter and implemented its advice, try the questions again.

- I believe in myself to always follow the correct path, even when challenges try to upend me.
- I have a clear sense of my purpose in life, and make decisions that are true to it.
- I know what I'm passionate about and I make sure my

lifestyle – in terms of my job, pastimes and adventures – reflects my passions.

- I understand that my mind has a profound influence over my well-being and I take steps to ensure my thoughts serve me.
- I make time every day to pursue activities that make my heart sing.

THE NEED TO BELIEVE

Many people don't realize the profound influence of the mind in determining the state of physical health. The mind affects everything from our energy levels to our immune system. Think of the times when you're working too hard, under pressure or worrying – aren't those the times that make you most susceptible to sickness and disease? It's as though germs and toxins are secret agents waiting to wreak havoc within vulnerable, stressed-out bodies.

When you have self-belief – that is, when you are fundamentally at peace with and motivated by the way you are living your life and the direction you are taking, confident that you can achieve your goals – you inherently hold a positive energy that makes you strong, resilient and competent. You drive through barriers, shake off minor illnesses, and have the potential to reach beyond your expectations. So, if you want to live a life that is forever young, you have to have self-belief.

In fact, US developmental biologist Bruce Lipton goes one step further – he claims that having belief actually has a genetic expression within our bodies that changes our physiological well-being: "The question of age has been really not built into the genetics. It's built into our minds, our perceptions and our beliefs because its through the chemistry of our mind and brain and what we believe, that ultimately selects the genes and modifies the gene expression."

SELF-ACTUALIZATION AND BELIEF

In the 1940s, US psychologist Abraham Maslow identified that we have a hierarchy of five basic "needs". He believed that if we can fulfil all of these needs, we can live a meaningful, fully enriched life. The five needs, in order of importance (beginning with the most basic and ending with the most aspirational) are:

- physiological needs (for food, water, shelter and warmth); safety needs (for security and stability, and freedom from fear);
- belonging needs (for love and family, and friendship);
- self-esteem needs (for respect, recognition and a sense of achievement in life);
- self-actualization needs (for creativity and fulfilment).

In terms of living a life that you can believe in, it's number five – self-actualization – that I believe is key. Put simply, it's about identifying our true potential through identifying what drives us and gives our life meaning and then realizing that potential to the best of our ability. However, in order to make self-actualization possible, we need first to have fulfilled all the needs that come before it. That's okay – because already in this book you have learned the importance of nourishing your physical self and improving your sense of security, belonging and self-esteem through the many aspects of love. Now it's time to find out your greatest motivations in life – your passions and purpose.

PASSION AND PURPOSE

To have passion for something is to have an overwhelming – almost uncontrollable – belief in the value of that thing.

A passion is far more than a pastime; it drives you. We talk of "igniting" a passion – it is fiery and has energy that fuels you and drives you powerfully around obstacles that threaten to send you off course. Passion comes from within; it draws from your life-force and wells up inside of you as an untameable sense of *having* to connect or engage with something. For example, passion in a relationship is an all-consuming, unquenchable desire to be with that person. Passion for your work will take you beyond the nine to five, to achieve results that no-one else dreamed of, perhaps even beyond the reason of sleep or rest. Passion for a cause might drive you to perform acts in the name of that cause that defy logic and even common sense.

Purpose, on the other hand, is both the reason for something's existence and the sense of determination – the belief – that a person feels towards a particular aim or outcome. Your purpose is what you believe you came to Earth to achieve. It requires the level of energy that fuels a legacy.

So, what happens when we bring passion and purpose together? Passion can run riot without the direction of purpose; purpose can feel worthy or burdensome, without the energy and motivation of passion. Identifying your passion, and tempering it with purpose, empowers you to carve a meaningful future; a future filled with belief.

It sounds easy, right? But actually finding your passion and your purpose and following them without a hint of insecurity or doubt are among life's greatest challenges.

Removing doubt

In Secret 5: Love, we talked about the importance of self-love – of talking to yourself kindly, being gentle with your perceived failings and forgiving yourself when you feel you have done something wrong. In effect, self-love and self-belief go hand in hand. When you have self-belief you have the removal of doubt, and utter faith that the path you are taking is the right one.

So let's work out what your levels of self-belief (and doubt) are like now, then you'll know how to move on from that place in order to find your passion and purpose and head towards your goals with complete conviction.

Tune in to your internal dialogue – just like you did when you were learning to show yourself forgiveness (see page 118). Listen to your thoughts and your replies to your thoughts and consider whether they represent positive self-talk, or if they undermine you.

Now think of something you want to achieve this week, but haven't yet got round to. It doesn't have to be a big life goal – choose something tangible and measurable. Perhaps you started this week intending to run for 30 minutes every day (or every other day), but haven't managed a single session yet; perhaps you had intended to call an old friend, check up on a sick friend, or visit an elderly relative, but every day has passed and you've not made the call or visit. Now think about why – is it time pressure? Is it that you were worried you couldn't cover the run distance? Or, that you weren't sure your friends or relative would want to hear from you? How does not achieving that one simple goal make you feel? How differently would you feel if you'd managed it? What really stopped you? Was it really that you couldn't find 30 minutes in your day? (If so, go back and read Secret 2: Move!) Was it really likely that an old or sick friend, or an elderly relative wouldn't want your company? (If you really think so, go back and do the exercise in Secret 5: Love.) When you break those thoughts down, I doubt that any of them will stack up. The only thing that stopped you was that voice in your head.

So, now let's think about turning that voice into one with a can-do attitude. Start seeing challenges on your path to realizing your passion and purpose as opportunities – things that will help you learn how to overcome the obstacles to where you need to go. Start praising yourself when you notice a difference in your thought patterns, when you meet a challenge and don't let the voice in your head stop you from overcoming it. Soon you'll start, almost imperceptibly, to switch from putting barriers in the way of achieving your goals to opening doors that take you to them. Start celebrating the wins in your life, no matter how big or small. Just as self-love will bring more love into your life; positivity will help to bring yet more success.

So many people go from relationship to relationship, from job to job, from place to place, expecting to find happiness outside of themselves. Of course, there's nothing wrong with change, and sometimes it can be a blessing, a relief, or "as good as a rest". But the only change that really matters, that really makes a difference to whether you're living forever young, is the one that takes you from a negative mindset to a positive one, rich with self-belief. Your external world is a projection of your internal world. To live forever young, your mindset is the place where it all begins. There is nothing as powerful as a mind transformed to believe in the power of positivity.

FINDING YOUR PASSION

So, if you don't already know what your passion is, how do you find out? The first step is to try my passion test, answering the following questions. Answer each one honestly and fully. Don't put limits on your answers – time, money and commitments – as these count for nothing for the purposes of this exercise. You have a free rein to do or say exactly what you please. Write down each answer on a piece of paper – you may find that the questions have more than one answer each. That's okay. Write down up to three answers each time, if you like. For the last question, you can give as many answers as you like.

- *What makes your heart sing?*

Is there any one thing that makes you feel the tingle of joy throughout your whole body? That makes your heart want to leap from your chest and your whole face light up? I truly believe that happiness and passion walk hand in hand. Both lift your resonance to a higher frequency – making every cell in your body buzz with excitement. For me, it's the moment I see the sunrise over the crest of a hill or the swell of the ocean; or the look on people's faces as I see they have connected with me and are on the cusp of transforming their lives; or the energy in the room filled with people whose lives are changing right before me.

- *What activities just flow from you, as though you were born to do them?*

For some people, this might be playing the piano or violin, or singing – when the sound that comes out of you (whether through your fingers or voice) is so pure and natural and effortless, and yet fills you and everyone who hears you with joy. It needn't be something artistic, though – perhaps you are a natural long-distance runner, gymnast, mother or teacher; perhaps you are a natural raconteur. Try to think of things that you know some people dread or find difficult or are wary about, but for you feel effortless.

When I was growing up, for me it was gymnastics. I remember working (and playing) at it for hours and hours, and always coming up with different moves and crazy stunts, creating routines to music. Gymnastics has always been, for me, creative, fun, energizing. It's my passion.

- *What would you never tire of doing?*

Often this is something really creative that changes or transforms every time you do it or discover something new about it. For example, your passion might be a subject you could read a hundred books about and still be hungry to learn more; or something that you create once (a painting, a photograph, a sculpture, a particular recipe dish) and then want to create again and again, refining until you reach mastery, but never tiring of trying. It's the thing that makes time slip away – before you know it, you've been doing it for hours and could still do more.

• *What would you do for free?*
This is an interesting question, because often the thing we'd do for free is quite different from the thing we choose to do for our job. But what if you could marry the two? How amazing would life be then? Perhaps you would choose to spend your time teaching children, or helping those less fortunate than you, building houses, decorating houses, fishing, ice skating, acting, singing or painting. Whatever it is, this is a key question, because I think there are jobs out there that can match most people's "If only I could spend my days..." More on this shortly.

• *On your deathbed, what activity or experience would you never want to add to the sentence "I wish I'd tried..."?*
If you were to live a full life – a life that is boundless, with infinite possibilities, a life during which every time you would usually hesitate or say no to something new you said yes instead – what would your strength, passion, determination and drive empower you to do?

Starting right now, you're going to make a list of the experiences that are on your bucket list. You have your whole life ahead of you – aiming to fulfil each of the items on your list will give you purpose, inspire your passion, and help you to keep looking forward, living forever young.

Look back at the lists you've made in response to my questions. Can you see any similarities or resonance between each? Is there overlap? Are there patterns in the sorts of things you're choosing to resonate with? Are there harmonies? If you can, group some of your answers together (it doesn't matter if there aren't any groupings – this is just a question of tidying things up, so that you have clarity for where your heart lies). Now you have your lists, you know what really inspires you, ignites you, motivates you. It's time to bring more of those things into your life.

PASSION AND YOUR FREQUENCY

I believe that all the cells in your body vibrate at a certain frequency. There is a resting frequency for healthy, happy, steadfast people and it is best understood and monitored by how generally good you feel consistently. However, when I talk to people about their passions, their optimism rises to the surface and their energy levels clearly increase. The more of this energy we can harness, the more we can create in life. This shows just how important it is to identify and value what makes us highly emotionally engaged. Passion increases your voltage, which in turn also bolsters your immune system helping to protect you from illness and disease. The highest vibrations and energy of all occur when people feel the emotion of love – imagine what might happen to your longevity when you combine your passion with love.

When you shift your attention from negative self-talk or pessimism to focusing on pursuing your passion, you automatically give your cells the opportunity to vibrate at a higher frequency. That means that you start to live your life in this fundamentally positive state – even at a cellular level. In this way the potential for wellness is with you long into your old age.

CREATING SPACE FOR YOUR PASSION

Imagine a world where everyone could wake up and do exactly what made their hearts sing. What a beautiful world that would be! In my view the perfect world is one where your passion becomes your daily life – where work stops being the thing that earns you money and instead fulfils at least some elements of your passion. Work should never be a chore, it should be a privilege that you get to experience. Something you're grateful to get up to every morning.

Find the tools, get the skills, find ways forward – you could do all those things or any of them, if you allow your passion to fill your consciousness.

Now, I'm not so unrealistic as to think that you can all ditch the day jobs, risk the mortgage, leave the kids to forage for food and abandon all creature comforts so that we can follow our passions. Of course, we have responsibilities, but just imagine if you could identify your passion or passions and then translate elements of them into what you do for a living, or find ways outside of your working life to fulfil them. Let's say that you find that you are passionate about music, food or dancing. Start an orchestra at your local school, or invite parents to join a band that meets every Saturday for an hour, just to jam with any instruments that come along. If you want to cook, get a stall at a Christmas market and sell pickles, jams or home brew; throw a dinner party once a month and treat it like a restaurant night; once a week take inspiration from a food trend and create your own dish that really nourishes whomever you share it with – not just in terms of ingredients, but through the love and *passion* you used to create it. If you want to dance – dance! Join a local salsa group, learn ballroom or simply spend an hour a day with the music turned up loud, and bust some moves. Make time to bring your passions into your life. You do have time. I promise you, you just have to choose passion as a priority.

The decisions we make about how to spend our time are determined by what we value most. So if you want to create change in your life and make room for feeding your passion, all you need to do is connect to what you value most. For example, let's say that you value your family above all else and your greatest passion is sailing, take your kids on a sailing course in the holidays (you don't have to charter a yacht – start in little sailboats on a lake so that you can learn, laugh and love together). Or, if you place most importance on the time you have for meditation, and your passion is dance, learn moving meditation or whirling dervish, or use dance steps as a focus for mindfulness.

Furthermore, stop saying "should" and start saying "must" in relation to your passions. If you can't combine your passions and your job, schedule time for pursuing them – put them in a diary or on a calendar and prioritize them. Your passions need to become non-negotiable.

In my case, I prioritize self-love above all else, but my passion is to spend as much time with my family as possible. Although self-love is now something I practise every day, I also spend time at retreats, alone, in order to reconnect with myself and give myself the time I need to resonate in pure vibrational tones. But why would I spend time at a retreat alone or with my partner, looking after myself without my family, if my passion is the pursuit of excellence in my commitment to my family? This is how I see it: every time I look after myself I make myself a better person – a more positive and connected person. Then, when I am with my family, I am the best version of myself I can be and that positivity resonates among all of us, increasing the vibrational frequency of our family get-togethers.

**You can accomplish anything you believe in.
So the most important thing is to believe, and
once you believe, it is.**
Guy Obolensky – inventor and entrepreneur

WHAT IS YOUR LIFE PURPOSE?

So, you've identified your passions and you've learned how to make space for them. But at the start of this chapter we identified that to be able to live with utter self-belief, our lives need purpose, too. Anyone with a deep religious belief will possibly associate their purpose with serving their God. Doctors, nurses and other medical practitioners might align their purpose with extending and saving lives. Charity workers and volunteers may see their purpose in life as helping those in need. Many people will consider their purpose to be accumulating wealth to pass on to their children. Maybe our ultimate purpose is simply to ensure the survival of our own species. My purpose, as I see it at this time in my life, is to pass on the word about keeping our bodies and minds as healthy as they can be while helping people to really live their dreams. Maybe you've not yet worked out what your purpose is and that is totally okay. In all honesty, you may never find, or be able to articulate or define, your life purpose because it changes at different stages in your life, like chapters in a book.

What if your purpose was to make sure that your body serves you well throughout your life? What if you learned to harness energy so you can create anything your heart desires? What if you could learn to respond to life with a powerful love so that you are always living in the moment, as the greatest version of yourself? Everyone can live *with* and *on* purpose, being your best self with a vitality that keeps you young and is contagious. As Confucius said, "Choose a job you love, and you will never have to work a day in your life."

Your purpose as a foundation of rock

A philosophy professor once stood before his class. When class began, wordlessly he picked up a large empty jar and proceeded to fill it with rocks of about 5cm (2in) diameter. He then asked the students if the jar was full. They agreed that it was.

So the professor then picked up a box of small pebbles and poured them into the jar. He shook the jar lightly. The pebbles, of course, rolled into the open areas between the rocks. The students laughed. "Now is the jar full?" asked the professor. "Yes," came the reply. The professor picked up a box of sand and poured it into the jar. Of course, the sand filled everything else.

"Now," said the professor, "I want you to assume that this is your life. The rocks are the important things – your family, your partner and your health. They are anything that is so important to you that if it were lost, you would be nearly destroyed. The pebbles are the other things that matter, like your job, your house and your car. The sand is everything else – the small stuff. If you put the sand into the jar first, there is no room for the pebbles and the rocks. The same goes for your life. If you spend all your energy and time on the small stuff, you will never have room for the things that are truly important to you."

He went on, "Pay attention to the things that are critical to your happiness. Play with your children. Take time to get medical checkups. Take your wife out dancing. There will always be time to go to work, clean the house and fix the waste disposal. Take care of the rocks first – the things that really matter. Set your priorities. The rest is just sand."

So what do we take away from this? I think it's telling us that our life's purpose is defined by the things (and people) that are most important in our lives. So, the next time you find yourself getting stressed out over being five minutes late for a meeting because the traffic is bad, or wanting to tear bits of paper into shreds because the printer broke down – put things in perspective. Did a member of your family fall ill? Have you just been told that you have a serious disease? Have you lost your partner? No, no and no. If you allow the grains of sand in your life to negatively affect your energy, your vibrancy, you aren't carving out your life according to its main objective (to fill it with rocks). Instead, you're allowing the grains of sand to adversely affect your health and (because you'll likely not be much fun to be around) your relationships.

It's a true story

I do love what happens to people once they've really experienced how living forever young makes them feel. I once worked with a movie producer who was struggling with a documentary she was making. By learning how to believe in herself and how to shine, she started on a new path in life and completed her movie in a very different way, with a different outlook, because she had a new clarity and was focused on serving herself and others at the highest level. Her new confidence enabled her to do all the business deals needed to make the movie a success. Her documentary is now winning awards all around the world and she is glowing by simply allowing herself to shine wherever she goes. She now lives with the balance and happiness we all deserve.

WRITING A PURPOSE STATEMENT

So, now that we've established that family, health and that special someone are the rocks in your life, how can we translate that into a purpose statement that summarizes the essence of why we should believe in our lives?

In an essay, speech or thesis, a purpose statement sets out the aims of the work. It summarizes them in a single sentence or short paragraph so that the reader or audience knows exactly where the writer or speaker intends to take them. If you can do this for your life, based on the need to prioritize the "rocks" in your life, you will immediately have something tangible and direct to aim for.

Try it now: Write a purpose statement*

Now it's time to have a go at writing your own purpose statement along those lines, so get a piece of paper and a pen and off you go... Here are some top tips:

- make it believable;
- make it personal;
- make it achievable;
- make it fun;
- make it honest;
- make it enjoyable.

It can be as short or as long as you like – it is personal to you, after all – but around 100–200 words is usually a helpful length. Get your ideas down as quickly as you can – try to make your writing instinctual. You can always refine your early draft. Once you have written it, look at the tips above and see if it fulfils these criteria. And check in with your statement regularly – so you can be reminded of it and recommit to it along your journey.

Remember, finding your purpose is a way you can give real meaning to your life with a clear direction – it is about believing that what you set out for yourself is worthy of you and believable for you, that it is authentic.

My purpose statement goes something life this: "The purpose of my life is to nurture my health and energy through eating foods that are kind to my body, practising exercises that help me to stay fit, supple and strong, and protecting my emotional, mental and psychological well-being by tuning in to my inner thoughts and feelings and making them resonate at a frequency as high as it can be. It is to nurture my family through kindness, respect, consideration and connection, never taking them for granted, checking in with my immediate family at least a couple of times a week and with my extended family once a month, making sure they know I am always here for them whenever they need me. It is to give myself openly and freely to my relationship – opening my heart, releasing jealousy and anxiety, and letting love resonate between us without suspicion or insecurity; it is to give my partner freedom to be herself in order that she feels truly, naturally connected within our bond. And to make things fun and joyful so I can share what I'm learning to help people transform all around the world."

THE MAGNETISM OF BELIEF

When you are living your passion with purpose, it lights you up inside and everyone who comes in contact with you can feel that light. When you are living your purpose, you feel the desire within you to get out and *do it* – no more of that sitting around at home considering what you'd prefer to be doing, actually *doing* it – and that naturally connects you with other people, emotionally, physically and spiritually.

Living your life with passion and purpose, and full of self-belief, is not a solo experience. It is infectious and inspiring. My general observation is that the people I work with who follow their passion on a daily basis are less susceptible to illness, have more vitality and are generally happier. I believe we all have a life purpose. Whether we are living it or not is another thing. But once we start to live it, health and wellness naturally follow. It's like all of a sudden you have the sense that you have a clear, powerful belief in life that automatically extends to living longer, younger and with more vibrancy. People will identify you as someone who is authentic, true; and they will naturally draw to your magnetism. Those who live with belief are fun to be around; they hold themselves confidently and openly – others want to share in that energy, which in turn generates more connection, more positivity and more resonance. And that means more longevity.

NOW YOU CAN BELIEVE

Believing in yourself is an attitude, believing in yourself is a choice. Most people are slowed or weighed down in life by their perception of themselves. That being the case, every encounter and experience has the risk of being weighty and cumbersome rather than filled with joy and positivity. However, if you follow the advice set out in this chapter, identifying your passions and defining your purpose, then embedding them into your life so that you truly live by them, your life takes on an authenticity – every moment has meaning and you're heading for a goal that is truly meaningful to you. It's at that point – when even if you don't know your life purpose itself, but you feel it and have made every moment count – that you start to believe in yourself and in the world's own energy.

With that belief you'll strive forward, and in that way life stretches out before you, longer and more fulfilled.

LIVING FOREVER YOUNG
TOP 10 TAKEAWAYS: BELIEVE

• Identify your passions – what are the pastimes, activities, experiences, events and relationships that make your heart sing?

- Identify your purpose – in the short term and the long term – and write a purpose statement. If you can't yet find your purpose, don't worry – if you live by your passions, your purpose will reveal itself in time.
- Believe in the potential for greatness that lies within you – and then set out to be great.
- Recognize when something lights your fire – could it be a passion?
- Recognize that improvement comes from within – only you can make things better, more authentic, more energetic, more joyful.
- Let go of self-doubt – it doesn't serve you and holds you back. Think instead that even if you bruise your knee, your skin will not only heal on the surface but also deep within. Always believe in your own power for self-healing.
- Keep with the positive self-talk – it raises your frequency and makes your body vibrate with positive energy.
- Always aim for the greater good in your actions – think of the ripple effects of your life.
- Look after the important things first – don't worry about the small stones until you've taken care of the rocks, or the sand until you've nurtured the small stones.
- Believe that you have all you need inside of you to create everything and more in your own life.

OVER TO YOU

Now that you've read the bulk of this chapter, it's time for you to choose how exactly you are going to make the secrets of believing *your own* by integrating them into your daily life. So…

- Close the book and consider the ways in which you would feel most able and happy to start putting this chapter's suggestions, or any other believing-related ideas of your own that you have, into practice.

- Then take a pen and notebook or piece of paper and write down the three, or five, of these ways that you most like the idea of really committing to, and that you feel will not only be really useful for you, but also achievable and sustainable. For example, you might commit to focusing every morning before you get out of bed on the belief that you are ready to live your best day ever; sticking up little notes in suitable places around your home to remind you what great gifts you have to share with the world; or share a secret passion with a friend or loved one and watch them come alive as they lock into your energy, enthusiasm and self-belief.

- If the thought of three, or five, things overwhelms you, just start with one – baby steps are the best way to go and as long as you keep up what you have started you'll soon find momentum building and you will want to, and be able to, do more.

- If you need a little help and encouragement to get into this decision-making zone, try the "Lost in Music" technique on page xxi to set you on your way.

- Then read your chosen action points out loud to yourself – and make an inward commitment about how, when and where you're going to start putting them into practice – as of this week, or even *today* if possible. Feel free to write these practical details beneath the action points if you feel it will help you stick at them…

- Now use this list as your personal guide to enhancing the "Believe" section of your life-balance wheel, coming back to the list any time you feel the need to revise it or add to it…

✎ WHERE ARE YOU NOW? (PART 2)

Once you have been using the above list of action points for about a month, it will be time to assess how things are going. So – remember that list of statements you rated at the start of the chapter? Well, read and rate them again (I've listed them below, so that you don't have to flick back).

Please score the following questions for believing on a scale of 1 to 10, with 1 being "not at all true for me" and 10 being "completely true for me".

- I believe in myself to always follow the correct path, even when challenges try to upend me.
- I have a clear sense of my purpose in life, and make decisions that are true to it.
- I know what I'm passionate about and I make sure my lifestyle – in terms of my job, pastimes and adventures – reflects my passions.
- I understand that my mind has a profound influence over my well-being and I take steps to ensure my thoughts serve me.
- I make time every day to pursue activities that make my heart sing.

Your ultimate aim in terms of a score is 40 or above – an 80 percent plus result that shows you have this secret nailed and are really using it to help you live forever young. Keep pushing yourself, however, and do what you can to avoid being complacent and slipping back into bad habits.

If you're implementing the takeaways and practising your chosen action points/techniques, I hope you'll see that your score has improved since the first time you did it.

If you're not quite where you want to be, return to the "Over to you" section in order to revisit your key action points and ensure that they still feel relevant to you (see page xx for more advice on revisiting and reassessing your goals).

After you have been practising your new "Believe" techniques for a while, don't forget to revisit your life-balance wheel at some stage (see page xxii) to keep track of progress in terms of how you feel in this area of your life. This will help you to acknowledge your achievements and to keep making further progress. The more you shade in every segment, the bigger the steps you are making along your path of living forever young!

SECRET 8: LEARN

Learning is in every day. Each time you have a conversation with a friend, you learn new thoughts and ideas, details and nuances. Every time you meet a challenge in your job, your relationships, your parenting, you learn ways to overcome those challenges, and often learn about yourself, other people, your capabilities and your strengths and weaknesses. Every time you read a newspaper or watch the news, you're learning something new about the world. Every time you write an email or a letter, or explain something to your children or a friend, you're learning ways to articulate yourself. Learning is in everything. This chapter is about the importance of learning in myriad ways through your experiences and your pastimes in order to keep your mind forever young.

To stimulate your mind is also to nourish your body. As we learned in the Introduction to this book, the mind, body and spirit are intimately connected. In this chapter, we'll look at how nurturing your mind can help to keep you feeling and being young, long past the notion of "old age". We'll look at ways in which to keep your mind being stimulated and fresh; and tactics and exercises that will keep pushing you to extend and build on your mental capacity, to keep your thinking fluid, balanced, creative and energetic. We'll look at how positive mental energy staves off the onset of mental illnesses, including depression and even dementia, and how that also keeps us physically active by giving us a general joy for life.

But, before you begin, let's look at where you are with your learning, right now.

WHERE ARE YOU NOW? (PART 1)

Please score the following questions for learning on a scale of 1 to 10, with 1 being "not at all true for me" and 10 being "completely true for me". Note down your score. Then, when you've completed this chapter and implemented its advice, try the questions again.

- I have discovered the best ways in which I learn: listening, reading, watching or experiencing.
- I stimulate my mind daily with challenges and experiences that help me to learn more about myself and those who surround me.
- I learn more about myself by pushing myself to the limits of my comfort zone every day.
- I share my experiences with others and enjoy listening to other peoples' stories.
- I have a thirst for knowledge – I probe and question every new thing I learn until I fully understand it.

THE NEED TO LEARN

You're probably wondering how in the world my pursuit of knowledge has anything to do with my passion for longevity, health and happiness. It's simple: as I said in the opener to this chapter, to stimulate your mind is to nourish your body. Some of the best money I've ever spent has been on educating myself.

This connection between the state of our minds and the health of our bodies is so evident to me now that it seems almost *too* obvious to require an explanation. However, I know there was a time when I didn't see the connection and I had to

stumble gradually over the insights in order to see the truth.
I hope that if you are where I was back then, I can make the
process of understanding quicker for you.

Eastern mind–body wellness techniques (including yoga
and t'ai chi) draw upon the powerful ways in which your body,
thoughts, emotions and behaviour can directly affect each other.
If you've been practising your *pranayama* yogic breathing from
Secret 1: Breathe, you'll already have discovered how closely
connected the state of your mind is to the state of your body.
With all that controlled expansive breathing, you'll have noticed
how your circulation becomes rhythmic, your lungs absorb
oxygen to their fullest capacity, and your mind – simultaneously
– becomes quiet, collected, calm and yet powerfully alert. If
you've felt this unison between the calming of your mind and
body, you've felt the mind–body connection.

Interestingly, though, it's not just ancient Eastern practices
that believe in the health benefits of nourishing the mind: the
ancient Greeks also believed that our minds and bodies are one.
They hypothesized that physical fitness was a manifestation of a
fit mind and that a fit mind would result in a body that strives to
be fitter. Throughout his writings, the ancient Greek philosopher
Plato emphasized the importance of bodily exercise for
developing the mind. His ideal was the harmonious perfection
of the body, mind and psyche.

Through all those ancient teachings, Eastern and Western,
and through my own experience, I believe that keeping your
mind flexible, challenged and creative will not only keep you
mentally young and able, but physically young and able, too.

YEARS ON YOUR MIND

Your brain began to form inside your mother's womb a mere
16 days after you were conceived. How mind-blowing is that?

175

Over the next weeks, that early, budding brain turned over on itself, became tubular (we know it as the neural tube) and started to control the function of foetal growth. By the time a foetus is eight weeks old, there are enough neurons (nerve cells) and synapses (fiery communication ports) throughout a baby's tiny body that messages can zip around to control movement and cell division. Amazing.

After birth, in the first three years of life, the brain develops more rapidly than at any other time. In fact, by the age of three, a baby's brain is three times heavier than it was at birth. That's because this is the time of life when we learn more than we ever will – when everything is new, from the shape of our mother's face to the smell of her milk and the sights, sounds and smells that surround us at every minute. As we take on new information, the brain and nervous system form new neurons and new pathways between neurons until we have about 1,000 trillion of those connections by the age of three. The brain and nervous system are so clever that over the course of our lives they reform connections constantly, linking together experiences and memories to create a network that is unfathomable in its intricacy – and yet, apparently, using only about 10 percent of our brain's full capacity. Incredible. Imagine what could be possible if we could only tap into the power of the other 90 percent!

We often hear people talk of the brains of children being like sponges – they seem to absorb information easily, effortlessly. They also tend to learn joyfully and with wonder. I think there is a connection between the two. If we treat the world with wonder and joy, as if seeing it through a child's eyes, learning itself becomes playful, which opens our minds to new experiences. In my own experience, information that I hunger for, and that I love learning, sticks.

Which brings me on to what happens as we age. During adulthood, I think of the brain as going through a stage of petrification – it starts to harden against learning, things become more difficult to retain, there's more interference and more distraction. Life, for many, starts to lose its wonder. With the onset of responsibility come stress, doubt and fear. That's not to say we don't still have the capacity to learn throughout our adulthood – I believe that we do! And that's what I want to bring back for you.

At its most practical level, we learn as we progress through our careers, or develop expertise at family dynamics, or at communicating with others as we meet new friends, colleagues and partners throughout our life. But the questions we have to ask ourselves are: do we still love learning? Do we still treat the world with wonder? Is learning contributing to our mental, physical and emotional well-being? Is it helping us to live forever young?

If the answer to any of those questions for you is no, then keep reading.

Your memory

Contrary to popular belief, there's no inevitability about forgetfulness. Although many of us think we are slowly finding it harder to remember things, and that memory loss is an irreversible sign of ageing, actually it's more a question of layers. The more stress layers there are on top of the memories (whether for facts and figures or personal history), the harder the memories are to find. But, as long as you keep exercising your brain in inspiring, creative and active ways, and reducing the layers of stress that lie over all the wonderful, amazing information and skills you store, there's every reason to believe that your memory can serve you perfectly well long into old age. In fact, the brain is making new neural pathways all the time, connecting and reconnecting experiences and memories as you go about your daily life. If a pathway lies dormant and unused for a while, it naturally dies away, while new pathways are forming. But, if you keep reinforcing your memories, and using your brains pathways, they can stay strong. Just think: use it, or lose it.

> **Your ability to actually derive the highest grade information comes from the present moment. The present moment contains the entire future in the making.**
>
> Thom Knoles –
> Maharishi of Vedic meditation

KEEPING YOUR MIND FOREVER YOUNG

Earlier on we talked about the importance of recapturing some of your youthful exuberance in your learning. In order to do this, there are several steps I'd like to take you through. First, we'll look at identifying what kind of learner you are – that is, the ways in which learning most fires your imagination. Then, we'll look at practical ways that you can apply each learner type to keep your brain active and youthful.

What kind of learner are you?

First, a definition. The National Institute of Adult Continuing Education (NIACE) Adult Participation Survey (2015) says that "learning can mean practising, studying or reading about something. It can also mean being taught, instructed or coached. This is to develop skills, knowledge abilities or understanding of something. Learning can also be called education or training. You can do it regularly (each day or month) or you can do it for a short period of time. It can be full time, or part time, done at home, online, at work, in another place like a college or at live events and retreats, etc. Learning does not have to lead to a qualification."

SECRET 8: LEARN

The key there is that learning can be done anywhere, anytime. You don't need to change your schedule for this. You don't need to spend an arm and a leg. For some of you, it might be as simple as listening to talk radio shows with interviews with great thinkers, podcasts, politicians or authors; for others, it might be doing a weekly pub quiz. It might mean going to the park to sit down with a green tea and the latest historical novel. It may be learning the steps to a dance routine at a local salsa class. You may be interested in learning how to play the guitar. It could even be a date with your *National Geographic* magazine during your lunch hour. For me, learning is buying a bunch of audio books that I can pop on while I'm driving, or sync onto my iPod for when I'm doing some fun exercise. I also read health, fitness and longevity research. It's truly amazing how my concentration improves when I've exercised my "concentration muscle" by reading something! We all learn in different ways and we all have unique interests – find out what yours are and go after them!

Since the 1970s there have been various different hypotheses about "learning styles", fundamentally boiling down to the fact that some of us learn more readily in certain ways than others. For example, one system suggests that people fall into one of seven different categories of learner: visual, aural, verbal, physical, logical, social and solitary. If you're a visual learner, say, you might assimilate knowledge more easily if you see it in pictures (are you the kind of person who found mind maps the most useful method for revision, perhaps?). An aural learner is most engaged when information comes in auditory form – that is, you learn best when you hear and listen. I have a particular love of audio books and will often listen to them while I'm travelling or working out as mentioned above. I find that that really gets my brain firing. Verbal learners are words people – they learn through reading, speech and writing. A physical learner uses the senses and particularly the sense of touch as a means to assimilate information; or might learn best while they're on the move. Reasoning and argument works for someone who is a logical learner, while a social learner is more likely to enjoy group work, and a solitary learner prefers to study alone.

All that sounds very formal to me – and I know that formal education (including school!) doesn't suit everyone. When I say that I think we have to use our brains to live forever young, I don't necessarily mean that it's time to give up the day job and go back to school. What I mean is that if you can identify how you best like to learn (and you may think you fall into more than one category – for me, I would say I prefer both aural and physical learning), you can try to stimulate your brain in those ways in your daily life. Let's take each learner type and look at a few creative and inspiring ways to keep your brain active.

Visual learners – paint, draw, visit a gallery

The Japanese art of calligraphy is a form of meditation (called *sho do*): the calligrapher focuses the mind fully on every brush stroke, bringing a sense of alert calm, while becoming mindfully immersed in the activity of painting. If you are a visual learner, taking up a practice that encourages your creativity while also stilling your mind and extending your learning (your creative craft) is just about the perfect combination.

Alternatively, make time each week to visit a gallery or local art store. Check your local newspaper for art trails. Each time you look at a painting really study it – consider the brush strokes, the nuances of meaning in the images (what does the sky tell you, the expressions on faces, the poses and so on; can you see any symbolism?). As long as you are thinking about what you are doing, you are fully absorbed in a task, which means you're learning.

Aural learners – sing, jam and listen

I think there is nothing more liberating than turning the music up loud, singing and dancing like a demon. We touched on this in Secret 2: Move. This time, though, it's time to turn music into a medium for learning, for extending your neural pathways in new directions and proving to yourself that there is a rock star (or opera star or orchestra star) within you.

The obvious way to learn through music is to learn an instrument – or to take up again an instrument that you stopped playing as a child. Guitar, piano, flute, drums, even the plain old recorder – find an instrument that you love and start playing. You don't have to have lessons, just play in your own time. With every note you're making new neural connections and you're giving your mind a focus that will send energy pinging through your whole body. If nothing else, spend ten minutes a day in glorious voice. Just sing freely.

But there are other ways to learn and listen, too. Do as I do and download audio books on topics that interest you and listen to them in the spaces – while you're travelling to work, running, at the gym, cooking dinner. That's the great thing about information that's going through your ears – you can plug yourself in and just let those synapses start firing.

Verbal learners – keep a diary, write a novel, learn a language

There are so many options for a verbal learner! Writing and talking about subjects that fire your imagination are the perfect ways to keep the brain active. For a daily task, write a diary, making a note of the new experiences, your emotions and your interactions. Keep a memory jar – each day summarize three key things that happened on a small piece of paper and pop it into a jar. At the end of the year you can go back and read each piece paper, consolidating those memories to keep your brain firing. Alternatively, if you have the time, write your life story, a chapter

– even a paragraph – at a time; or talk to an elderly relative and start writing theirs.

If you have time, try learning a new language, or offer to give a speech at your local school about your job or an exciting adventure you went on. Offer to cover story time at your local nursery. Verbal learners get so much mental agility out of any activity that involves the use of words – whether written or spoken.

Physical learners – engage your senses

A particular smell or sound can awaken a memory of a particular time in your life, especially if the experience occurred at a time when you had a heightened emotion, good or bad. Think of times when a particular memory has been kicked off for you just by smelling a specific scent or hearing a distinctive sound or tune. Physical learners experience the world with all their senses, and consolidate learning if they learn while they're active.

Your five major senses – sight, sound, touch, smell and taste – are powerfully connected to your memory, and using them as a means to engage your brain is easy – you can do it every day and at every moment. Right now, run your hand over the page of this book – how does it feel? Really, how does it feel? Describe it to yourself as if you were telling a friend who had no sense of touch at all – be as detailed as you can be. A friend of mine always smells the pages of a book before she starts reading it – what do these pages smell like? Don't just think "paper", try to describe them in unusual ways, using unexpected comparisons (like buttery leaves, like freshly cut wood, like béchamel sauce laced with cinnamon…).

If you're a physical learner (and even if you're not), try to treat the world with this level of wonder – like a child discovering something for the first time and yet without all the vocabulary to describe it, which means making comparisons that might seem unusual, but somehow get the message across. Engaging your senses fully in your daily life will help you to form strong, lasting memories.

Finally, physical learning might mean using your body to discover something new. Learning the steps to a dance routine, or the moves in a fitness class engage the parts of your brain involved in coordination and memory – forming bridges and connections that otherwise wouldn't exist. Furthermore, learning physical activity gets you into the present moment – while you're remembering the steps, you are fully engaged in now. And that's good for your mental space and your spirit, too.

Logical learners – discover science

If you're a logical learner, look to the sciences for inspiration. Can you see the patterns in the stars? In numbers? There are thousands of books out there with fascinating stories of how scientists came to the conclusions of the meaning of life that we take for granted. Or, discover science in your home. Take something apart and put it back together again – your bicycle, your electric toothbrush, a fidget spinner. Work out how things work. And don't forget sudoku – the perfect puzzle for a person who likes numbers!

Social learners – share with others

Whenever I am asked to share what I already know with others, I try to paint images, tell stories and invite my audience to share mental, physical, emotional and sometimes spiritual experiences with me. When appropriate I always invite and encourage the audience to participate and contribute their experiences, too. These sharings are so powerful.

I always come away from my presentations or my live events with more knowledge and insights that I went in with. I love to learn from my audiences. Think about this – what if you could learn something new from every person you connected with? How would that help you to grow and reshape your reality?

How many times do you hear an argument being made lucidly by an apparently well-informed commentator and slightly, or even totally, change your mind over the rights and wrongs of a situation? Then listen to the counter argument and change it right back again? I know I often do. It doesn't mean you are weak-willed or uncommitted. It means you are learning that the truth is sometimes elusive and you frequently have to ask many questions, and hear and share many viewpoints, before you can come to a conclusion that serves at the highest level.

So, if you're a social learner, how do you bring all those benefits into your everyday life without spending time on retreats or going to conferences? There are so many ways! Start a discussion group at your house, join a book group, simply arrange to meet friends to find out how they think, or share a predicament, or discuss a topic of interest during your lunch hour. Don't shy away from talking. Try treating every social interaction as if it is an opportunity to learn something new – about the world, about yourself, about others.

Solitary learners – take some quiet time

So, you're a solitary learner? Wow! So many opportunities for stimulating your brain and getting those neurons firing in personal ways that suit you! Let's start with meditation. Spending just 10 to 15 minutes every day in quiet contemplation, reflecting on your thoughts, acknowledging them and then filing them, or (if they don't serve you) letting them go, is enough to be able to still your mind, consolidate your learning and memories from the day, and nourish your spirit. Do it! Make time every day: just for you and your neurons.

Alternatively, take time each day to do something that stimulates your brain in an active way – a crossword, sudoku, writing a diary, playing solitaire, painting (if you're also a visual person), knitting, baking, reading a book on your most passionate topic (see Secret 7: Believe) – all of these are ways to engage your learning, to keep your mind active and young.

LEARN, THEN LEARN SOME MORE

I firmly believe that for learning to really mean something, for it to resonate through all your body's cells, as well as making new connections in your brain, when we need to hit upon something that really interests us (it could even be your passion), we have to keep probing so that we learn, then learn some more.

Try to resist ever saying to anyone, or even thinking, "I already know that." If you've made that decision before you've digested what you're being told, you're not fully engaged. Every piece of text, every piece of information you hear might have a nuance of meaning or a new perspective that you've never encountered or considered before. Everything is worth your full attention – in itself that's simple mindfulness.

Of course, you might not agree with or understand everything you read or hear – and that's good, too. Question everything that seems out of kilter and keep questioning until you're convinced of the answers. All the time you're probing and discovering, you're keeping your brain working.

Then, use your knowledge creatively. If you like, start a website or blog about what you're learning – and invite comments from others. See what happens, what more you learn, and keep experimenting. Being creative with what you learn, using it to begin new pursuits and new ventures, is in itself energizing. It will help to build your confidence, which will feed your thirst for more learning, more understanding. That's the thing I love most about learning – the possibilities are infinite, the energy is limitless.

An enquiring mind is a healthy mind; so let's stay interested and curious.

WHERE CAN I START?

Next time you find yourself waiting at the doctor's surgery, or have a spare 10 minutes while you wait for your kids to come out of school, set up that time as a learning hotspot. Pull out a book or a magazine, write in your journal, listen to a podcast, complete a crossword puzzle, watch an inspiring video on your phone. Use those pockets of time that so often get lost in our lives. Even if you just close your eyes and learn to watch and embed your thoughts as they travel across your mind, you're using the time wisely.

NOW YOU CAN LEARN

Learning stimulates the mind, which keeps the mind young, and learning is in everything – every interaction, every experience, every conversation, every adventure. Furthermore, mental agility – through games and puzzles and learning new subjects or skills – has been proven to stave off the onset of typical "old age". I believe that while the mind is young and active, the body remains young and active, too. And vice versa. By consciously acknowledging and developing what and how you learn into your new everyday life, you will be letting this secret play its part in helping you live forever young.

Finally, always remember the sense of wonder that children have when learning about the world around them – be a kid yourself, so you can Keep Improving Daily!

LIVING FOREVER YOUNG
TOP 10 TAKEAWAYS: LEARN

- Consider how your mind and body are connected – when your mind feels strong, you are able to find strength in your body.
- Take up a new hobby or recapture an old one and discover (or rediscover) the joy in getting better at something.
- Stimulate your mind daily with books, audios, videos or puzzles. Or find an activity that has always eluded you and crack it!
- Connect learning to your passion (see page 156) so that learning becomes pure joy. Think of ways to make learning personal to you.
- Never stop learning – if the first certainty in life is death, the second is that there is always something to learn from the world around you.
- Use listening as learning – remember that everyone you meet has something to teach you. Learn something new from each person you connect with – every day.
- Watch children at play and learn from their creativity and freedom. Try to recapture some of that spirit of abandon in your own life and see what new truths it unfolds.
- Learn from your mistakes – acknowledge them, then let them go and move on without a backward glance. Life is all experience and learning, even when things go wrong.
- Share your learning – the buzz and energy of collective learning raises us to be better than we thought we could be.
- Use the spaces in every day as learning opportunities – even if it's just learning to watch your thoughts as they move across the screen of your mind.

OVER TO YOU

Now that you've read the bulk of this chapter, it's time for you to choose how exactly you are going to make the secrets of good learning *your own* by integrating them into your daily life. So…

- Close the book and consider the ways in which you would feel most able and happy to start putting this chapter's suggestions, or any other learning-related ideas of your own that you have, into practice.
- Then take a pen and notebook or piece of paper and write down the three, or five, of these ways that you most like the idea of really committing to, and that you feel will not only be really useful for you, but also achievable and sustainable. For example, you might commit to learning something new every day while you're doing something else (that is to say in the spaces of your life, using no extra time, such as popping on a podcast while you're travelling or cooking), or signing up to a course in an area that you've wanted to try for ages, or try turning a negative into a positive by focusing on a mistake you've made in your life and thinking about what you learned and took away from it going forward.
- If the thought of three or five things overwhelms you, just start with one – baby steps are the best way to go and as long as you keep up what you have started you'll soon find momentum building and you will want to, and be able to, do more.
- If you need a little help and encouragement to get into this decision-making zone, try the "Lost in Music" technique on page xxi to set you on your way.
- Then read your chosen action points out loud to yourself – and make an inward commitment about how, when and where you're going to start putting them into practice – as of this week, or even *today* if possible. Feel free to write these

practical details beneath the action points if you feel it will help you stick at them...

- Now use this list as your personal guide to enhancing the "Learn" section of your life-balance wheel, coming back to the list any time you feel the need to revise it or add to it...

📝

WHERE ARE YOU NOW? (PART 2)

Once you have been using the above list of action points for about a month, it will be time to assess how things are going. So – remember that list of statements you rated at the start of the chapter? Well, read and rate them again (I've listed them below, so that you don't have to flick back).

Please score the following questions for learning on a scale of 1 to 10, with 1 being "not at all true for me" and 10 being "completely true for me".

- I have discovered the best ways in which I learn: listening, reading, watching or experiencing.
- I stimulate my mind daily with challenges and experiences that help me to learn more about myself and those who surround me.
- I learn more about myself by pushing myself to the limits of my comfort zone every day.
- I share my experiences with others and enjoy listening to other peoples' stories.
- I have a thirst for knowledge – I probe and question every new thing I learn until I fully understand it.

Your ultimate aim in terms of a score is 40 or above – an 80 percent plus result that shows you have this secret nailed and are really using it to help you live forever young. Keep pushing yourself, however, and do what you can to avoid being complacent and slipping back into bad habits.

If you're implementing the takeaways and practising your chosen action points/techniques, I hope you'll see that your score has improved since the first time you did it.

If you're not quite where you want to be, return to the "Over to you" section in order to revisit your key action points and ensure that they still feel relevant to you (see page xx for more advice on revisiting and reassessing your goals).

After you have been practising your new "Learn" techniques for a while, don't forget to revisit your life-balance wheel at some stage (see page xxii) to keep track of progress in terms of how you feel in this area of your life. This will help you to acknowledge your achievements and to keep making further progress. The more you shade in every segment, the bigger the steps you are making along your path of living forever young!

SECRET 9: COMMIT

If you commit fully to your purpose, your passions, your views and your activities, you unlock your potential for greatness. When people come to my conferences or retreats, the thing I ask from them right at the start is to commit to the process they are about to undertake – to play fully with everything I have planned for them. I want them to commit with a positive attitude that reflects their belief in their own ability to live forever young.

In this chapter, I want to explore the notion of commitment and how it affects your longevity. For example, how the way in which you commit to your purpose, your goals and your relationships, and the attitude with which you commit, can all have a positive – or negative – effect on your well-being. I also want to look at the ways in which commitment might be challenged in your life, and how to develop a natural state of positivity, flexibility and resilience, in order to steer yourself around any obstacles that might make your commitment waiver. Where you commit yourself needs a conscious, considered decision – after all, the one thing you can't get back in life is time, and every moment matters.

But, before you begin, let's look at where you are with the notion of commitment right now.

WHERE ARE YOU NOW? (PART 1)

Please score the following questions for committing on a scale of 1 to 10, with 1 being "not at all true for me" and 10 being "completely true for me". Note down your score. Then, when you've completed this chapter and implemented its advice, try the questions again.

- When I set my mind to something, I rarely get distracted from my cause.
- I am able to visualize the end result in order to commit to an action, and I do so in as much detail as possible.
- I am thankful – rather than fearful or doubtful – when opportunities come my way and I grab every one without a moment's hesitation.
- I approach new tasks or challenges on my journey with a positive attitude.
- I refuse to give up on something that I want, even when I encounter obstacles or someone tells me that my goals are futile.

THE NEED TO COMMIT

To get the best out of anything in life – whether that's a job, a relationship, one of my retreats – you have to commit fully to it. On a retreat I need full commitment from my participants because I ask them to examine and then redesign their lives. Not only do they need to commit to that process so that they get the best – and the right – answers out of it, but also so that they commit to their lives going forward. You can't fake that kind of commitment because it requires total, daily action.

BELIEF AND YOUR COMMITMENT

If you don't fully believe in the goals you're setting for yourself, you can't fully commit to them. Having full commitment to your beliefs, passions and purpose is so important because there are lots of ways in which life – with its temptations and frustrations – will try to throw you off the path. Let me give you an example.

It's a true story...

The owner of one of Britain's biggest juicing companies came to one of my retreats. During the experience, he identified that a goal for his life going forward was to live at a higher level of being – to stay balanced through stress, and to really tune in to his inner frequencies, responding to life's curve balls with composure and resilience. He spent his time committing himself to his goals. When I called to check on him a few weeks after he'd got home, he told me that he was feeling very proud of himself. He had been let down by a major supplier. The "old" him would have lost his cool – taking out his stress on his team and his family. The post-retreat version, though, remembered his commitment. He engaged fully with the problem, dealt with it himself and found a solution within an hour. Throughout he was calm and effective – he responded in his greatness, not as a victim. He had come away from the retreat committed to the belief that he could change his behaviour pattern – and he did it with great results that he said he couldn't have imagined were possible before.

All the world's greats – artists, musicians, lovers, businessmen – have achieved their greatness from their commitment to their goals. One of my coaches once asked me, "Do you want to be a jack of all trades and master of none? Or do you want to live with mastery?" I chose to commit to mastery – and I believe I can achieve great things if I commit to that goal every day. Be prepared to win at your craft day after day. If you are lacklustre in your commitment to your beliefs you will lose your focus, and the curve balls and distractions in life will take you off course. When you commit, you're already a massive step forward in getting the deal done.

COMMITMENT AND ATTITUDE

There are two ways in which your attitude towards committing yourself can dramatically change how likely you are to be distracted from your path. First, you need to develop a feeling of thankfulness for your life and your opportunities; and, second, you need to enter into the spirit of your commitment with utter positivity.

Let's start with being really thankful. Please don't pass on this, because being thankful for every opportunity, every life challenge, every breath, is essential if you're to commit to your life's path. Here's how to develop an attitude of gratitude.

Visualize your future

If you can visualize your future with your goal already in place, you can be thankful that whatever life threw at you to get there – you did it. If your goal is physical (a family, a beautiful home, an inspiring job), you can visualize that end-game in all its glory. If your goal is more intangible (like my client – being calm in the face of disaster), play out the scenario in your mind with everything as you wish it to be. Imagine how thankful that future self is for everything that's happened, and everything that got you precisely to that point. And be thankful for achieving your aim itself.

Give thanks on waking

When you wake each morning, before you get out of bed, offer thanks for the little things in life. Begin with being grateful that you're alive and for your own mind and body. Give thanks to your eyes for all the wonderful things you see. Be grateful for your ears for all the wonderful things you hear (from the sounds of the birds, to the rumble of distant traffic, to the sound of your partner's breath beside you). Be grateful for your beating heart; for your hands that can touch, hold and soothe; for your feet

194

and the places they take you. Be thankful for the room around you, the comfort of your bed, the warmth of the covers and the softness of the pillow. Look around you and be thankful for all the trappings of your life that you see even before you've left your bed.

Of course, you don't have to stop at the little things – you can keep spreading your gratitude outwards to your loved ones, to the wider world, even to the universe.

When you enter each day positively, consciously giving thanks in this way, your attitude is enough to quieten some of the day's natural resistance. You start out with the aim of living that day as the best version of yourself. In your heart you expect that the day will bring you the greatest opportunities, and you'll welcome each of those opportunities believing that they have something of value to offer you. Valuable things don't need to offer resistance.

It's a true story...

I want to make a confession: I used to struggle with being grateful for small things because I was chasing the big things in life. Then, when life wasn't serving me, when I was floundering around, uncommitted to anything in particular, ungrateful for what really mattered and unhappy, I made some changes. I realized that I had so much to be thankful for within myself and around me in those I loved. I noticed that when I gave thanks for the small things, the big things came more easily. Showing my gratitude, and really feeling it, commits me to striving forward with more love, passion, joy, excitement and strength. Being grateful for the small things helps me to commit to my goal of serving others, and helping them to become the best versions of themselves.

Give thanks for your food

The notion of saying "grace" before every meal might seem old-fashioned, but in fact pausing to reflect on the nutritious bounty in our life is an important way to remember that, as we commit ourselves fully to our lives, we have to remember and appreciate all the things that sustain us – physically as well as spiritually and emotionally. To do so is empowering and energizing.

You don't have to give thanks out loud – just try to get into the habit of it in your head, if you like, saying a private thank you for the food that is about to nourish your body. Say thank you for its growth and its preparation, and for those you have the opportunity to share it with. Savour every mouthful, be present to the experience of eating and socializing around the table (put your phone away!). There's more on this in Secret 3: Nourish (see page 66).

Give thanks for your health

Whatever the reality of your physical health – even if you are suffering in some way – you are here, your heart is beating, your eyes are seeing, your brain is interpreting. Be thankful for all the health that you have and that you are striving to improve. Be thankful that you have the means to evaluate your health and to improve it. Give thanks for where you are and commit to your journey for improving your well-being.

Be thankful for nature's health-givers – the sun, water, oxygen. Next time you feel the sun on your skin, the wind on your face, the rain on your skin, the air on the tip of your nose, be thankful.

Give thanks for your relationships

Thank those closest to you for caring about you every day, and appreciate all the relationships you have (at work, among friends, as well as within family). The more committed to your life you become, the more you'll start to identify greatness in all those around you – and you'll appreciate how they share that greatness with you. Show your appreciation: leave little notes on pillows, or in a handbag or wallet; leave a message of love on an answerphone, flowers on a doorstep, or a card on a hall table; make a colleague a cup of tea or arrive at the office with a tray of treats. Show how thankful you are and in doing so commit yourself to all your relationships, from those you love to those you work with.

In addition, look out for the little acts of kindness people show you. I bet there are more than you think there are, when you start looking. Did someone open the door for you today? Or help you carry your shopping? Perhaps someone in the street offered you a smile as they walked by. My mother taught me that saying thank you costs nothing, but the payback in terms of continued kindness is often manifold.

Commit with positivity

There is no doubt that creating a positive mental attitude is essential in your attempt to commit fully to your life goals. Any niggles or doubts corrode commitment because they are like rusty cracks in the ship that makes the journey.

I can't think of any form of greatness in my life that has come to me without some kind of challenge. I have learned, time and again, that there's no point in backing away from a challenge when it faces you – you have to hit it head on, no matter how enormous it seems. When I was told I would never walk again, I could have let that force me to turn away from my dreams of being an acrobatics champion. Certainly, at the start of the diagnosis I was in a dark place. But slowly, and with some powerful soul-searching, I realized there was still greatness within me. Instead of letting my accident finish me off, I faced the challenge. Although becoming the English Sports Acrobatics Champion seemed impossible at the time, in 1992, less than two years after my accident, I did it. That journey – the one that took me from my place of despair to reaching my goal – taught me invaluable things that I now share at my live events, helping others to move past the obstacles that life throws at them and reaffirming their commitment even in the face of apparent disaster.

Every significant religious, mythological and historical figure – from Jesus to the Buddha – has followed the hero's journey. For example, for Jesus there was fasting for 40 days and nights; for the Buddha there was a life of austerity before reaching Enlightenment. Part way through a hero's journey towards greatness something happens that challenges the path. By working through that challenge (sometimes multiple challenges – think of the Greek epic hero Odysseus and all the crazy obstacles that he came across, from having his ship lured onto the rocks by singing sirens to having his crew turned into pigs by a witch), reinforcing their commitment to the cause, every hero realizes that what lies within is stronger and more powerful than anything life might throw at us. You have so much more inside you than you realize. So, whatever else you commit to in your life, always commit to your greatness, because that will conquer all.

> **The second we give ourselves permission to become immortals, we start setting goals that are beyond our life. If we have a goal beyond our life, we live longer.**
>
> John Demartini – author and
> human behaviour specialist

COMMITMENT SHAKES

No, this isn't a reaction to your partner saying they want to get married! Rather, it's an acknowledgment that no matter how committed you think you are to your goals, life is unpredictable and sometimes cruel. It's perfectly normal for those of us with even the strongest commitment to have a bit of a wobble every now and then. So what attitudes do you need to cultivate to deal with the commitment shakes?

Simple: flexibility and resilience.

Flexibility

Japanese Zen Buddhism talks of water flowing around rocks in the stream. The image is a metaphor for us to be free, flexible and flowing in order to navigate our path around the obstacles that life throws at us. In the Japanese Zen garden, gravel or sand represents water and is raked in curving patterns around rocks. Next time you go on a walk, try to find somewhere that has a free-flowing stream or river. Watch the movement of the water as it tumbles over debris on the riverbed. Little islands rising in a river might force the water to change course – but it always flows towards the sea. In other words, the destination is always the same.

In yoga, we use physical flexibility to free up the flow of subtle energy within the body, improving strength, vitality and balance. The flexibility of the body mirrors the importance of flexibility in the mind to enable open understanding, creativity and problem solving.

Of course, being flexible isn't just about obstacles. Even if the goal remains the same, the path you take towards it might need to change depending upon all manner of things in your life. It is very important for you to review your purpose/goal along the way and to be flexible and committed enough now and then to tweak the steps you take to get there. That doesn't mean changing your mind, or giving up, it means responding to your circumstances in order to get the best possible outcome for your purpose. In simple terms, think of a soccer match – both teams are aiming to win. At half time, one team is two goals down. In the dressing room, they have a team talk, make a few adjustments to their positions, and go back out onto the pitch with the purpose that's always been there – to win. This time, with a few tweaks to the team formation, things go well, and they score three goals in the second half and win. It's not how we start out that dictates the end result, it's how we finish.

Resilience

It sounds easy when you say "just flow around the obstacles in your way" – but, of course, it's not always that simple. When I thought I would never return to the gym again, the only things that kept me going were the firm commitment to getting better, and the resilience to pursue my quest to become a champion even when that goal seemed far out of reach. I had the vision, the belief and the unshakeable faith that I could make it work.

Try it now: Building resilience*

Here's an exercise to help you to cultivate that resilience when you need to meet an obstacle head on.

- Picture in your mind a time in your past when you were challenged and you let the challenge get the better of you – perhaps backing down in spite of yourself, or coming away from it feeling totally defeated. It might be a difficulty you had at work, or something more personal – perhaps in a relationship or with your children or other members of your family. Think of something that really knocked you out of kilter.
- Using all your senses, create that scene again. What was the event? Who was there? Where were you?

»

What sights and smells and sounds were around you?
Really conjure up the image of the scene, but try not
to attach any emotion to it – think of yourself as an
impassive observer.

- Now, start eavesdropping on the event, but not
only can you hear what's going on, you can also hear
inside your own head. Listen to what you're telling
yourself – are your words supportive or defeatist?
Are you telling yourself to face this setback head on
or to give up? Are you speaking kindly to yourself,
or disappointingly?

- Remember you're an impassive observer – and
not only that, you have the stop button. Visualize
yourself stopping the action. Rewind the scene and
start it again. Get back inside your head and replay
the event, only now with a positive self-talk – this
time you have the ability to turn things around;
to show that you have the resilience to face the
setback and turn it to your advantage. See yourself
overcoming the challenge with confidence, and
growing into more of your potential. Capture how
it feels to be that strong. Be proud of yourself –
you have the strength and resilience to overcome
any challenge life throws at you. Recapture this
visualization whenever you need to remind yourself
just how strong you are.

FINDING SUPPORT

Every life journey is our own. However, this doesn't mean that
we don't need the odd travelling companions along the way. In

fact, friends and loved ones – supporters – can be essential to ensuring our commitment remains firm. Your supporters are people who hold you to your highest standards and believe in you to do the things you believe in. Spend five minutes now writing a list of people in your life who fulfil that role for you. Think carefully – these are your unwavering champions, and although they may love you unconditionally, they also expect you to be true to yourself and to others. These are the true friends and family who will tell you straight when you fall, but also pick you up and dust you off. If you're very lucky, you'll have more than a few people on your list, but you are lucky enough if you have just one. Cherish them – they are few and far between. In my life, my mum has given me enough support for an entire army. She is the only person who has been through all of my challenges with me and each time she showed me the qualities and skills to help me believe that I could pull through. She didn't care whether I was facing a major physical challenge, a relationship challenge, a money challenge, a health challenge or a business challenge, she always believed that I would not only come out of it, but I would emerge a better person. I'm eternally grateful to have that support from her. I can't even imagine where my life would be without her belief in me.

Now, spend five minutes making a list of people who try to draw you from your path. Perhaps they undermine your achievements, belittle your life goals, or in some other ways (small or big) make you feel that your life's purpose is unworthy of their respect. For example, they might try to pull you backwards in your progress (perhaps literally leading you astray, or putting ideas in your head that make you doubt yourself). These are the people you need to shake from your life. They don't serve you and their counsel is not worthy of you.

And don't forget that every time you give someone else support in the truest ways, you invite that level of support in return. What you send out in the world comes right back to you.

SECRET 9: COMMIT

MAKING SACRIFICES

It's a cliché, but it's true – nothing in life is truly without
consequence. Commitment sometimes needs sacrifices. If you
are to truly to commit to something, it's likely you will need
to shed, ignore or sideline something else along the way. What
are you prepared to sacrifice in the name of your cause or the
pursuit of your goal? What are you prepared to sacrifice to live
forever young?

My decision to go back to acrobatics after breaking my
back was a big one that I knew needed my full focus and
commitment. My Bulgarian coach at the time was really clear
that I had to sacrifice all other distractions in my life: girls, other
work, study, partying. At the time, letting go of those things
wasn't easy. However, making my decisions polarized what was
truly important to me, what I was truly hungry to achieve. I
know from my own experience and from coaching other people
that the hungriest among us are usually the ones who find the
ways to make things happen against the odds.

So, what's stopping you achieving your goals – what
do you need to let go of? Could it even be laziness? Or
procrastination? Is it a person? Or a bad attitude? What do you
need to strip away so that you can focus on your goal and truly
commit? Every single, great person I know has made sacrifices.
Keep evaluating and keep stripping away what doesn't serve you.

MEASURING AND REWARDING
YOUR PROGRESS

Before we leave this secret for now, I want to tell you how I fully
endorse a system of reward. There's nothing like a bit of self-
congratulation to remind you that it's worth staying committed
to your cause.

To this end, it's important that you find a way to measure your progress towards your goal. Try breaking down your goal into stages. When I was aiming to become a champion, I set myself clear mini-goals that I could celebrate along the way. My celebrations weren't necessarily elaborate, but they were enough to make me feel good.

For example, a reward could be as simple as an evening in front of the TV or with your favourite novel, free from distraction; or a chance to sit in your favourite park and just let the world pass by. A hug from a friend, a high five, an indulgent slice of your favourite cake – all these can be little ways to tell yourself that you are doing more than okay, you're doing great. It doesn't matter what the reward is, as long as it feels good.

During my retreats, I consistently give rewards, praise, thanks, trust and respect to the participants at each stage in their journey. Each time we meet a mini-goal and celebrate it, a barrier goes down and the next stage of the journey opens up. Each time we come closer to our true selves, free from uncertainty and doubt and even more committed to our purpose.

NOW YOU CAN COMMIT

It's time to commit to your greatness, your relationships, your goals, your wonderful, beautiful *life*. Being truly, fully invested in your life is the only way to ensure that whatever life throws at you, you take it as an opportunity to be something better than you thought you could be. Committing in everything we do unleashes limitless potential from within. It sends that light (the one we learned about in Secret 6: Shine) outwards and turns every challenge into an adventure. Think of life as full immersion – you're in it, from the tip of your toes to the top of your head – go with it, live it and commit to it. Trust me, the rewards will be endless, but I have to warn you of some serious side effects: if you do this, you will start to look and feel younger!

LIVING FOREVER YOUNG
TOP 10 TAKEAWAYS: COMMIT

- When you begin an adventure, consider where you want to go and commit to the journey – do this as a visualization if it helps you.
- Be thankful for the air that you breathe, the sights you see, for waking and sleeping, and for love. When you're thankful you're showing the world that you're committed to it being a better place.
- Show positivity in all your endeavours, no matter how challenging. Don't let challenges throw you off the path – flow around the rocks in the stream.
- Give yourself permission to be flexible, when necessary, to adjust to changing situations.
- Be steadfast and resilient – tell yourself you are strong, feel that strength and show that strength.
- Cherish your core supporters and show them that you appreciate them.
- Be prepared to let go of people or situations that distract you from your goals.
- Reward your progress in small ways – every success is worthy of a cheer!
- Embrace life with love, passion and purpose.
- Look out for the little acts of kindness from the universe and others. They will reinforce how right you are to commit to your path.

OVER TO YOU

Now that you've read the bulk of this chapter, it's time for you to choose how exactly you are going to make the secrets of good commitment *your own* by integrating them into your daily life. So…

- Close the book and consider the ways in which you would feel most able and happy to start putting this chapter's suggestions, or any other committing-related ideas of your own that you have, into practice.
- Then take a pen and notebook or piece of paper and write down the three, or five, of these ways that you most like the idea of really committing to, and that you feel will not only be really useful for you, but also achievable and sustainable. For example, you might think about the things, physical or emotional, that are holding you back and make the decision to come to peace with them and let them go into the universe, or take stock of where you are on your journey to achieving one of your life goals and think about the next active steps you can take to achieving it, or even slow down and take some time to celebrate all you've achieved in your life so far and how proud those achievements make you feel.
- If the thought of three or five things overwhelms you, just start with one – baby steps are the best way to go and as long as you keep up what you have started you'll soon find momentum building and you will want to, and be able to, do more.
- If you need a little help and encouragement to get into this decision-making zone, try the "Lost in Music" technique on page xxi to set you on your way.
- Then read your chosen action points out loud to yourself – and make an inward commitment about how, when and

where you're going to start putting them into practice – as of this week, or even *today* if possible. Feel free to write these practical details beneath the action points if you feel it will help you stick at them…

- Now use this list as your personal guide to enhancing the "Commit" section of your life-balance wheel, coming back to the list any time you feel the need to revise it or add to it…

✏️

WHERE ARE YOU NOW? (PART 2)

Once you have been using the above list of action points for about a month, it will be time to assess how things are going. So – remember that list of statements you rated at the start of the chapter? Well, read and rate them again (I've listed them below, so that you don't have to flick back).

Please score the following questions for committing on a scale of 1 to 10, with 1 being "not at all true for me" and 10 being "completely true for me".

- When I set my mind to something, I rarely get distracted from my cause.
- I am able to visualize the end result in order to commit to an action, and I do so in as much detail as possible.
- I am thankful – rather than fearful or doubtful – when opportunities come my way and I grab every one without a moment's hesitation.
- I approach new tasks or challenges on my journey with a positive attitude.
- I refuse to give up on something that I want, even when I encounter obstacles or someone tells me that my goals are futile.

Your ultimate aim in terms of a score is 40 or above – an 80 percent plus result that shows you have this secret nailed and are really using it to help you live forever young. Keep pushing yourself, however, and do what you can to avoid being complacent and slipping back into bad habits.

If you're implementing the takeaways and practising your chosen action points/techniques, I hope you'll see that your score has improved since the first time you did it.

If you're not quite where you want to be, return to the "Over to you" section in order to revisit your key action points and ensure that they still feel relevant to you (see page xx for more advice on revisiting and reassessing your goals)!

After you have been practising your new "Commit" techniques for a while, don't forget to revisit your life-balance wheel at some stage (see page xxii) to keep track of progress in terms of how you feel in this area of your life. This will help you to acknowledge your achievements and to keep making further progress. The more you shade in every segment, the bigger the steps you are making along your path of living forever young!

SECRET 10: LIVE

Finding a single word for this secret was tricky, until I realized that what I wanted to share with you boiled down to helping you create the right environment to *live* in. Your environment – the space in which you live – has a dramatic impact on your physical and mental well-being. We have already talked about the impact of the mind on the body. In a sense, your mind and body are your inner space, everything under your skin. Now, we can talk about your outer space, how the outside world you live in is having consistent effects on the way you look, on the way you feel and the way you live.

If you looked inside the cells of your body with enough magnification you will find mostly space – I found that pretty mind-blowing the first time I learned it. And think about this: if you look into your outer world you'll also see mostly space. How we choose to fill that inner and outer space defines our happiness, our strength and balance, our success, our resilience, our passions – all the secrets we've learned up until now – and, ultimately, how healthily we age. In this chapter I'll teach you ways to consider your life so that you can be sure to create an environment that is ready for you to fill with everything that serves you, giving you a vibrational energy that enables you to live forever young.

But, before you begin, let's look at both the physical and emotional space that you've created for yourself to live in right now.

✎
WHERE ARE YOU NOW? (PART 1)

Please score the following questions for living on a scale of 1 to 10, with 1 being "not at all true for me" and 10 being "completely true for me". Note down your score. Then, when you've completed this chapter and implemented its advice, try the questions again.

- I make choices that protect my health and the health of the environment.
- I have designed my home and lifestyle to nourish me spiritually, creating spaces where I can be at peace.
- I surround myself with people who support me in raising my game.
- I believe that everything I do and all the choices I make have consequences, so I make decisions carefully with a world view in mind.
- I frequently push myself beyond my comfort zones in life, and am fearless of failure.

THE NEED TO LIVE

There are two ways to look at your "environment". First, you can consider the environment you physically live in – that is, the air you breathe and soil you walk on, and also the home you create for yourself and the people you fill it with. Then, you can look at your inner environment – the spaces within yourself, in your head and heart, and your spirit, which together are so fundamental to your experience of living forever young.

THE WORLD YOU LIVE IN

Imagine you're a fish living in a fish tank. In order to stay healthy, you need your owner to regularly clean your water and oxygenate it so that you can breathe purely. What a happy fish you'd be. Now, imagine that you aren't that lucky. You're the fish who belongs to the owner who never cleans the water and leaves it to stagnate with a lid on the tank.

I wouldn't treat a pet fish like that, would you?

And yet, we are all fish swimming around in the goldfish bowl of the world. It's our responsibility to ensure that, if we want to live forever young, we need to create a world that is as free from toxins and pollutants as is humanly possible. And, when we can't make the change, we have to protect ourselves as best we can against the harm that those pollutants can cause.

Organic food

We've already talked about the importance of fresh and live organic food and how to increase it in your diet, so I won't go back over it here – but, if you haven't already implemented this secret into your life, please go back and read Secret 2: Nourish and take all the steps you can. Remember that what you put into your body in terms of food directly affects the health of all your bodily systems – after all, the food you eat feeds your body's cells.

Organic beauty

Living forever young isn't just about what we look like on the outside (and with a purer inner space, we'll naturally look and feel younger anyway), but products that we use *on* our body make a significant difference to how healthy we are, too – after all, skin is permeable. That means that what you put on it gets into your system, just as if you were ingesting it. If you've started to research what's going into your food, extend that principle to what you put onto your skin or in your hair, and even what you use to clean your house. Here's a simple rule of thumb: if you look at the ingredients on a beauty or cleaning product and you wouldn't eat them, don't put them on your skin or in your hair, or use them to clean your home (think of those particles flying about your airspace).

Today, there are myriad natural beauty products and lots
of information available about how to make really effective
cleaning agents using store cupboard ingredients. We don't need
toxins on our skin and in our home. We just don't. There is
another way.

Cleaner air
Think of all the places you go in a day and how many different
environments you find yourself in. Remember that poor old
fish, floating about in his dirty fish tank? Too much of our air is
just like that stagnant water – filled with nasties that find their
way onto and into our bodies, and negatively affect our health.

One emerging area of research is into the effects of air
pollution on skin ageing. In 2016, researchers in Germany
published papers suggesting links between levels of nitrous oxide
(which comes from car fumes in urban areas) and increased
incidence of age spots, rosacea, wrinkles and other blemishes in
people who are exposed to them every day. When you think that
London had emitted more than its annual nitrous oxide target
in just the first week of 2016, you can see that air pollution
is potentially a huge problem for living forever young. And if
that's the damage it's doing to skin – what's it doing to us on the
inside? For now, who knows? But I've no doubt that evidence
will emerge that pollution contributes to ageing in all the body's
cells, not just those on the outside.

Of course, the practical reality is that we can't all hide
away in the least polluted parts of the world, but we can take
steps to minimize our exposure. Try to get away from the city
and all its exhaust fumes as often as you can – weekend walks
in the countryside or time away in the hills or on the coast are
a good start.

Many cosmetics companies now claim to provide products
that protect against harmful pollutants in our atmosphere – but
don't swap one damaging influence for another. Remember

to look for natural products that don't themselves use harmful chemicals. Some research shows that vitamin B3 can help to protect the skin against pollutants in the atmosphere; while others suggest that the skin has its own protection in the form of its natural oils – so avoiding scrubbing away the top of layer of skin cells, and using just water rather than soaps that strip the skin bare might provide some resilience.

It's a true story

At one of my retreats in Spain, a lady came to me with eczema all over her body – she had suffered with the condition throughout her life. (I had suffered with eczema as a child, so I really felt for her.) I took her on a supercleanse. We worked through all her cosmetics and creams and lotions and took out anything that had any toxins in it. We worked through her mental and emotional stress, clearing her mind of the mental clutter that was causing toxicity in her body. We freed her mind using meditation; and used yoga and other fun movement processes to get her subtle energy flowing through her body again. We spent time on a juice fast together – clearing her system of toxins. On the last day of the retreat she approached me and showed me her skin. She was completely free from her eczema. Every part of her body was clear. It felt like a miracle – she'd never been clear before – and yet, in truth, with some guidance and support, she'd done the job herself and can use this wisdom for the rest of her life.

Detox living

If your life allows, I thoroughly recommend an annual detox retreat. There is no doubt in my mind that having a deep cleansing and detoxing experience each year creates a cleaner system that glows with youthfulness, energy and longevity. Full immersion in a guided detox environment is the kind of cleanse – a sort of annual service – that gets your body's energy flowing freely again.

LIVING FOREVER YOUNG

However, if that's not practical for you, here is a way to detox at home – try a three-day juice fast to totally cleanse your body. Although this sounds like you'll just be hungry for three days, I promise you won't. Aim for about 5 pints (2–2.5 litres) of mostly vegetable juices every day. See Secret 3: Nourish, page 57, for more details. And, it goes without saying, for the juice fast, use organic fruit and veg to ensure that you're getting the purest foods into your body.

My guess is that once you've tried this, you'll want to make it a regular part of your life, perhaps even having a juice fast once a month. It's a good idea to practise it first over a weekend, starting on a Friday morning, when you don't have three days of work ahead of you. And it can be a good idea to avoid driving, for example, in case you feel lightheaded. At the start of the process, you might get a headache, but this is just a sign that the detox is working. Once the toxins have started to make their way out, you'll feel better, lighter, younger and fitter.

Spiritual home

We've already touched on the notion of using safer cleaning products in our homes, but what about the more spiritual aspects of our external environment? What about the links between how we balance our homes and our quest for living forever young?

In the ancient Chinese art of Feng Shui, the home is believed to have an energy flow, just like the body. When something blocks that flow, the flow in the body is blocked, too. This leads to imbalance and stress. Rather like this ancient Chinese art, I believe that we all vibrate at a certain frequency. That frequency is reflected in our homes – and the higher the frequency, the healthier, more balanced and more youthful we will be.

The first and most obvious way to get some positive energy flow back into your home is to have a good declutter. Get rid of things that take up space, and are unloved and unused.

214

Clearing your space will clear your mind, too. Every time you pull something out of a cupboard, ask yourself if you really need it – when was the last time you looked at it? Could you live without it? The less attached you are to material things the more you will flow with life. And don't think of this as a "spring" clean – I suggest you do it four times a year, with the change of the seasons.

Another good way is "smudging", the ancient practice of burning sacred plants to clear negative energy from a space and to bless the new, clean energy flow. Plants such as cedar, lavender, pine, cypress, frankincense, sage or rosemary are thought to have cleansing properties. Invest in an essential oil burner and use the oils from some of these plants to benefit from their health-giving, cleansing properties. For example, lavender will create a calming atmosphere; peppermint will clear tension; palo santo or frankincense will clear your house of negativity; and precious rose is believed to increase the vibrational frequency of an atmosphere in a home.

Positive relationships

Our environment is filled with people. The US entrepreneur Peter Voogd once said that, "If you hang around five intelligent people, you will be the sixth…; if you hang around five idiots, you tell me what will happen." He also explained that he keeps closest ten most valued and trusted people: five of whom will challenge him to be better than he believes he can be, and five longstanding, reliable friends who nurture and support him and ask him to be no better than he already is.

What's noticeable about this close-knit circle is that it doesn't include people who don't have a positive influence over his life. We touched on this in Secret 5: Love, but it's worth saying again here that in order to create an environment that best serves you, that raises your vibrations to a higher frequency, surround yourself with people who have a positive influence in your life. Seek their counsel when you need advice; ask for their opinion when you need someone to give you a kind, but straight answer. If someone's presence makes you feel stressed or negative or anxious, remove them from your life. It sounds harsh, but it's your life – you have one shot at living it, so live it surrounded by people who encourage, support, love and challenge you in positive ways.

Of course, you can't just feed off those closest to you. In order for them to remain positive in your life, you have to give something back, too. My best piece of advice on this is always be true to your word. Follow through on your promises, live an authentic life that engenders the trust of others, especially those whom you value most. Support and be supported; love and be loved; catch a friend who's falling and be caught when you yourself fall (then enjoy getting back up to live a better life).

YOUR INNER ENVIRONMENT

Inside and outside are intimately connected. Everything you experience outside of yourself – the physical, practical ways in which you live that we've talked about so far in this chapter – influence your inner space, too; and vice versa. So, how do we make sure that our inner environment is as healthy as possible? How do we ensure that it serves us to be the best version of ourselves we can be, to live forever young?

Live as if everything is connected

The really crazy thing about living forever young is that all our energy, all our vibrations are interconnected. That goes for the vibrations of a tree, of your home, of your neighbour, of your lover, of your own self. Even the blades of grass on which you walk. Everything is connected in a web of energy that spans the universe. That means that if we raise our own vibrations, we can increase the vibrations of all the connections that we have around us. Mind-blowing. That's why I want you to think about what energy you send out into the world, through all the secrets up until this point. Because if your energy is positive, clean, purposeful, powerful, focused, full of love and authentic, you'll send energetic vibrations out there to spread all that positivity, creating an environment that only has a positive influence right back at you, on your own inner space.

Do you remember physics lessons when you were taught that ripples will bounce back when they hit the bank of a pond? Well, that happens with you, too. In order to live at a higher frequency, we have to make sure we're sending out higher-frequency ripples so that higher frequencies bounce back. Even if they lose some energy on their journey, fundamentally they are made of positivity, of goodness.

All the information that your senses pick up from the outside world in the form of frequency gets into your body and then filters up to your mind. How you respond to those vibrations is entirely within your control – that's why we've learned the arts of passion, resilience and positivity over the course of this book. If you take those frequencies and make something worthwhile of them, you can live a life that has no such thing as "failure". Instead it has only opportunity to create something better, for yourself, others and the place you live in.

Incidentally, as a bit of an aside, I don't believe in failure. I believe that what others might see as failures are in fact powerful feedback on how to do something better next time. During my events I push all the participants outside of their comfort zones so that they experience what it's like to learn in this way. After one such event, one of my participants told me, "I live and work in a world where I'm putting so much stress on myself for making mistakes and getting things wrong. What I learned from this course is that it's okay to fail and that failing is an important part of growing and becoming more." When I asked him how the experience would transform the way he lives going forward, he replied, "I understand now that I will fail at things in the future. However, I can rationalize that before I even begin. I acknowledge that if I start at A and I want to get to Z, some of the letters I pass will seem to the outside world as failures on my journey. But, I know that each letter is just as important as each another because each has something to teach me. Now I can live each day giving my best and knowing there's something of value to learn, instead of focusing on crossing the finishing line and being frustrated if the journey there doesn't quite go to plan. Just to live in the present, appreciating every 'letter' on my journey from A to Z, is a simple but powerful way to get the most out of my life."

Your inner space is yours to fill. How you choose to fill it is entirely down to how you choose to live. There's no need for me to labour this point – it's simple and now that I've shared all these secrets with you, I know you'll understand me when I say: fill the inner spaces with positive energy and you'll feel positive; fill them with negativity, and you'll feel negative. Learning to live as you were born to live really just boils down to that.

> **It's important to set a goal for yourself, for your family, your community, your city, your state, your nation and your world for at least 100–120 years. If you do, you will live a long life.**
>
> John Demartini – author and human behaviour specialist

Try it now: Breathing in positivity*

Here is a visualization to help you get the balance right. All you need is five minutes and a quiet space to do it.

- Sit or lie comfortably. Close your eyes and imagine the trillions of cells that make up your physical body. Imagine them vibrating. Imagine the spaces in between them.
- In the spaces, imagine tiny particles of dust – these are the microscopic atoms of negative energy that you've collected in life. This negativity is bouncing into every cell as the cells vibrate.
- Now, take a deep breath in. As you breathe out, imagine clearing all those spaces – all those negative particles disappear with every out-breath.
- Breathe in again. This time you're breathing in positivity – the spaces fill with golden light. Remember the light that shines within you? You're cleansing yourself of all impurities and, instead, are filled with pure positive energy.
- Imagine your cells bathing in this positivity. Their vibrations in pure harmony and synchrony. You are free of toxicity and you are pure, positive light.

LIFE BEGINS OUTSIDE YOUR COMFORT ZONE

In simple terms, our brains are designed to protect us and to keep us surviving through whatever challenges we are faced with. Within this comfort zone, where it is safe, there is a part of us that isn't growing and expanding. So we are left feeling like we want more. When you start living forever young – as though you are hungry for life, and confident that you can live your dreams – this enables you to move outside of your comfort zone so that you can do more and become more. You have to see it and believe it to achieve it. When your brain tells you to retreat back into your comfort zone, you can encourage your spirit to override this and trust that you have what it takes to become the hero of your life.

Here are some ideas on how to move out of your comfort zone:

- Choose something that will have you push your boundaries – climb a mountain, sign up for a challenge, start a new class (exercise, language, pottery, whatever), get a life or business coach, the list goes on.
- Find an expert who has already walked a similar path and learn from them. Read about them, see them speak, whatever you can. This can be hugely valuable and save a lot of time and struggle as you'll get great tips and buckets of inspiration from them.
- Speak to trusted friends, family or a professional coach, and let them know of your new challenge and ask them to hold you accountable so that when you want to quit (and this is normal) they are there to give you the love and support to encourage you to carry on and reach your goal. Note: you have to be willing to take their advice and committed to taking the necessary action steps to stay on track.

Think of it like this – when you were a baby and were learning to walk, what happened? You fell over, a lot. But did you give up? Did people around you tell you you'd be better off not following that path, not learning how to walk? No. You kept going. Then, one day, you stood up and balanced yourself. What was the response from people around you? Nothing but a huge wave of positivity.

No one focused on the problem (you falling over) – it was all positive encouragement. Seeing you and believing you would stand up and walk one day. Everyone became part of the solution, including you, and no one bought into the problem. No one suggested you give up because you kept falling over. No one bombarded you with negativity. When you make mistakes in life, it's just the same as when you fell over while learning to walk. What if you could learn to just get on with it, and not complain or blame or worry about it incessantly, not become part of the problem yourself.

Once you've learned to be comfortable outside of your comfort zone, you will start to push the boundaries of life further and further, and you'll be amazed at what you can do. The sense of achievement you'll get from this will just boost you further – I really believe we all have the magic inside of us to be living forever young.

NOW THAT YOU CAN REALLY LIVE

So I really do hope that you're now inspired to remember how to live as the best version of you and to really enjoy your experiences in this crazy game of life that we get to share together. I'm so thankful for the challenges life presents me, because I know that it's getting me ready to live bigger, stronger, fitter and to reach the next level in life. I really hope this resonates with you so that, no matter what happens in your life, you live each and every day supercharged and superconnected. Every day you have the potential for adventure, for experience, for connection and understanding – you just have to cherish your environment (inner and outer) enough to truly *live* it.

LIVING FOREVER YOUNG
TOP 10 TAKEAWAYS: LIVE

- Respect your physical environment – make healthy, safe choices.
- Practise regular detox – both physically and spiritually.
- Cleanse your home – make it clutter-free and filled with love so that it feels safe, warm and inviting.
- Shed the downers in your life – fill your environment with people who challenge and support you in positive ways.
- Trust that life has a bigger vision for you when you are challenged, and strive to live up to its expectations.
- Tune in to the ripple effects all around you and respond accordingly.
- Don't let fear stop you – there are no failures, only lessons.
- Live in the present moment – the past and future are nothing and life is infinite.
- Fill your inner space with positivity – choose a healthy attitude at every moment.
- Just live. Life is great and so are you.

OVER TO YOU

Now that you've read the bulk of this chapter, it's time for you to choose how exactly you are going to make the secrets of good living *your own* by integrating them into your daily life. So…

- Close the book and consider the ways in which you would feel most able and happy to start putting this chapter's suggestions, or any other living-related ideas of your own that you have, into practice.
- Then take a pen and notebook or piece of paper and write down the three, or five, of these ways that you most like the

idea of really committing to, and that you feel will not only be really useful for you, but also achievable and sustainable. For example, you might decide to set reminders on your phone to pull you into the present moment a few times a day, so that you can check that what's going on will serve at the highest level for raising your quality of life; you might choose to make a conscious decision to always give your best in every situation; or you might decide to run through a list of all ten secrets in this book each morning to remind yourself what they are – and get ready to live your dreams in a body and mind you're proud of.

- If the thought of three or five things overwhelms you, just start with one – baby steps are the best way to go and as long as you keep up what you have started you'll soon find momentum building and you will want to, and be able to, do more.

- If you need a little help and encouragement to get into this decision-making zone, try the "Lost in Music" technique on page xxi to set you on your way.

- Then read your chosen action points out loud to yourself – and make an inward commitment about how, when and where you're going to start putting them into practice – as of this week, or even *today* if possible. Feel free to write these practical details beneath the action points if you feel it will help you stick at them...

- Now use this list as your personal guide to enhancing the "Live" section of your life-balance wheel, coming back to the list any time you feel the need to revise it or add to it...

WHERE ARE YOU NOW? (PART 2)

Once you have been using the above list of action points for about a month, it will be time to assess how things are going. So – remember that list of statements you rated at the start of the chapter? Well, read and rate them again (I've listed them below, so that you don't have to flick back).

Please score the following questions for living on a scale of 1 to 10, with 1 being "not at all true for me" and 10 being "completely true for me".

- I make choices that protect my health and the health of the environment.
- I have designed my home and lifestyle to nourish me spiritually, creating spaces where I can be at peace.
- I surround myself with people who support me in raising my game.
- I believe that everything I do and all the choices I make have consequences, so I make decisions carefully with a world view in mind.
- I frequently push myself beyond my comfort zones in life, and am fearless of failure.

Your ultimate aim in terms of a score is 40 or above – an 80 percent plus result that shows you have this secret nailed and are really using it to help you live forever young. Keep pushing yourself, however, and do what you can to avoid being complacent and slipping back into bad habits.

If you're implementing the takeaways and practising your chosen action points/techniques, I hope you'll see that your score has improved since the first time you did it.

If you're not quite where you want to be, return to the

"Over to you" section in order to revisit your key action points and ensure that they still feel relevant to you (see page xx for more advice on revisiting and reassessing your goals).

After you have been practising your new "Live" techniques for a while, don't forget to revisit this section of your life-balance wheel at some stage soon (see page xxii) to keep track of progress in terms of how you feel in this area of your life.

A FINAL LITTLE REMINDER ABOUT LIVING FOREVER YOUNG!

Congratulations! You have reached the end of the book and the ten secrets that I live my life by and encourage others to live theirs by too!

I hope with all my heart that you are now feeling much more full of energy and enthusiasm for life, "younger" in body, mind and heart, and that you feel brimming with ideas about the next steps to take to keep feeling more vibrant still…

Now, or some time soon, is a fantastic time to redo the entire life-balance wheel exercise from page xxii. This will allow you to see the progress you feel you've made in each of the ten areas, see how the balance of the different aspects of your life might have shifted, identify which areas you've made most progress in, and also decide which areas you feel you most need or would most like to work on. Remember to acknowledge your achievements – and, crucially, to keep believing in yourself. I truly believe that by following the advice in this book and in a range of other positive sources that inspire you, you will not only feel better and younger in yourself but also achieve great results in life, whatever that means to you. So I wish you every success on your continuing journey of living forever young!

Live Strong, Live Healthy, Live Long, Live Now!

With love, Skip

USEFUL RESOURCES

There have been so many amazing teachers and writers who have influenced me and my work over the years that I've decided not to try to sum them up here with a *conventional* list of books and articles, as I'm not sure I could do the broad range of inspirational influencers justice.

Instead I encourage you to explore the books and/or online content of the many inspiring people who I mention throughout this book for yourself, as well as exploring the work of any intriguing and inspiring teachers and writers you come across yourself, of course.

A curious and open mind is a wonderful thing and will help keep you "living forever young"!

I would, however, like you to have the chance to experience at least some of the practical exercises in the book in a more direct and potentially powerful way – as if you were at one of my live events.

As such (and as mentioned in the introduction to the book), I have created a range of additional free online material for you as a thank you for buying my book.

These can be found by going to www.SkipArchimedes. com/LFYadditionalresources and inputting your details so I can send you links to the recordings.

Below is a list of the main "Try it now" exercises that you will be sent audio versions of once you input your details (complete with their page references in this book):

- Three minutes of freedom (page 6)
- The power of water (page 75), including both...
  - Improving your inner flow
  - The mind as a pool of water
- Mindfulness meditation (page 95)
- Love yourself (page 114)
- *Ho'oponopono* (page 118)
- Inner light meditation (page 143)
- Write a purpose statement (page 165)
- Building resilience (page 200)
- Breathing in positivity (page 219)

You will also be sent a number of customized videos: one showing you a sequence of revitalising yoga poses to help you "live forever young", one guiding you through how to make a delicious green juice and one showing you how to whizz up a scrumptious superfood berry smoothie in a trusty blender. So I hope you find these both useful and enjoyable!

ACKNOWLEDGEMENTS

There is no way that I would have been able to share the powerful teachings within this book without all the teachers, students, clients, mentors and supporters that have helped to shape who I am today. I would also like to thank my friends and family who always believed in my vision to help people live a life of miracles by living forever young (as well as those who didn't believe). First and foremost, my dear mother, who has been by my side through all the ups and downs, and Dougy Fresh, who has been my wingman and a rock. Thanks to the Watkins team for joining forces to get this powerful message out to the world: Kelly, you rock; Judy, thanks for being strict with the content; and Becky, for keeping the magic alive on the pages. Also to Belinda, Deo and my Babygirl. It's a big team effort. Please forgive me if I've missed you out but you are all greatly appreciated. I love you all, Skip.

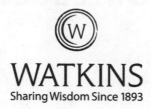

WATKINS

Sharing Wisdom Since 1893

The story of Watkins began in 1893, when scholar of esotericism John Watkins founded our bookshop, inspired by the lament of his friend and teacher Madame Blavatsky that there was nowhere in London to buy books on mysticism, occultism or metaphysics. That moment marked the birth of Watkins, soon to become the publisher of many of the leading lights of spiritual literature, including Carl Jung, Rudolf Steiner, Alice Bailey and Chögyam Trungpa.

Today, the passion at Watkins Publishing for vigorous questioning is still resolute. Our stimulating and groundbreaking list ranges from ancient traditions and complementary medicine to the latest ideas about personal development, holistic wellbeing and consciousness exploration. We remain at the cutting edge, committed to publishing books that change lives.

DISCOVER MORE AT:
www.watkinspublishing.com

Read our blog

Watch and listen to
our authors in action

Sign up to
our mailing list

We celebrate conscious, passionate, wise and happy living.
Be part of that community by visiting

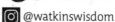

/watkinspublishing @watkinswisdom
/watkinsbooks @watkinswisdom